D1566239

Coordinating
THE
CHAOS

Through Birth and Burnout

D R. C HRISTY M ATUSIAK

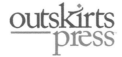

Table of Contents

Preface

Welcome to my labor of love. The material in this book has been on my heart for many years. As a holistic chiropractic physician, with every patient interaction I have, I'm sure I communicate much of this material one-on-one. I just knew that it was critical to share all I've learned over the last decade with as many families as I could possibly reach.

Truthfully, the content in this book was intended to be a weekend workshop, or a series of speaking events, where I envisioned empowering parents to step into the space of consciousness and learn about holistic healing. I had music, activities, reflections, and even food tastings planned! It was nearly ready to go, and I was excited to host my first one—and then it happened: The Coronavirus Pandemic 2020. Speaking events were a thing of the past, and I couldn't imagine doing this via Zoom, without the interaction and supportive environment of other people in the room. Without the ability to feed off other participants' energy, I was limited in how I wanted to proceed.

So, this book was born! It's always been my passion to support and care for new mothers and their families to create a loving and healthy household. My heart goes out to anyone who has had a baby in the last year, as I can't begin to understand the added challenges and uncertainty of having a newborn during a pandemic crisis. The "normal" resources, support, and social outlets were sorely reduced. It's possible you limited visitors for your own safety and comfort, while at the same time, the isolation and fear could have magnified the stress you were already experiencing. My heart goes out to all of you warriors!

Now, more than ever, we've realized the importance of our health. The better that we can protect ourselves with healthy choices, the higher our resilience and strength is against viruses and other challenges. More importantly, if we do this starting with our children as infants, they will grow up with fewer problems and health concerns. I'm excited to be here for you in your journey!

As a reminder, nothing in this book is intended to be a substitute for personalized medical care. My suggestions and thoughts presented here are with the understanding that this book is a platform for learning, and different situations require different interventions depending on the individual. Strategies discussed may not be suitable for every circumstance, and I encourage you to always consult with your trusted provider for the appropriate care for you and your family. This book is simply meant to encourage you to think critically and learn more options for your health and your life.

I'm so grateful that you chose to pick this book up. I'm filled with love and appreciation for the world of natural healthcare, where true healing is possible. Please enjoy the information I provided! If you ever have any questions, I include my contact information at the end of this book. I would love to meet you and support you if I can!

Yours in health,
Dr. Christy Matusiak

1

Motherhood Mayhem

Raising a child is a walk in the park...Jurassic Park, that is. ☺

I'm not a perfect parent. I've failed more times than I can count. And it is why I wrote this book.

I'd like to start by congratulating you on your new little bundle of joy! I bet you're feeling elated, energized, and excited for this journey! Blissfully happy and in the exact place you'd imagined! Waking up every day full of life and grateful for each moment! Knowing that this is *exactly* what you imagined when you dreamed of starting a family! ♥

Right?

Right?

...Not exactly? I'm sure you've heard it all—"Cherish these days, they go by quickly. The days are long, but the years are short. Hold her a little longer, rock her a little more. Read him another story, tell him a million more. Let him sleep on your shoulder, rejoice in his every smile. They are only this way for a little while...."

But let's get real. Motherhood is not all sunshine and rainbows. It's messy. It's ugly. It's not remembering when you last had a shower. It's not knowing the last time you slept. It's wondering if that smell of spit up is you or your baby. It's sometimes feeling like you're going to cry for no reason at all. It's feeling like a failure and full of doubt <u>every</u>. <u>single</u>. <u>day</u>. It's not knowing what day it is. It's wanting to return to work for some sense of normalcy and adult connection again, while at the same time never wanting to leave your baby. It's being overwhelmed and inundated with information, and yet still feeling desperate for more resources. You're trying to function, while healing from birth or C-section, and suffering from nursing issues and mastitis. Wishing your baby came with an instruction manual. You "google" sleep training, co-sleeping, starting solids, relationship self-help..." Maybe, you wonder if you're a bit depressed? But just press onward. After all, your baby needs you now. There is a completely dependent little human that is reliant on you for everything. It's not about you anymore. Suck it up and be the rock. You're a mom– your identity has forever changed. Does your partner even call you by your name anymore? Or are you just "mommy?"

I remember thinking—will I ever get back to <u>me</u>?! Do I even know who that is anymore?! How can I survive this?! Will I ever heal?! I'm in pain, and don't know what I'm doing! Will I ever go back to work? Will my body ever feel normal again? Will my partner and I ever connect again? I feel like I'm falling behind on life and losing myself. Everyone is expecting me to be radiantly happy, and I'm just feeling f@$%ed.

Then, our well-meaning friends and family want to come over and see the baby! They may bring food, and offer to help with dishes or something productive. But let's face it, they are there because they want to snuggle the baby. You're left feeling like you need to be awake, functional and entertain a guest, all while smelling like dirty socks, spit-up breastmilk and body odor. The baby cries, and they begin offering what they feel is support: "He looks hungry." "Want me to check her diaper?" "You should try holding him like this, or rocking her like this." And what started as a welcomed visit, ends with you feeling more alone and more like a failure than before.

What about the appointments with your baby's pediatrician?! They weigh and measure the baby, and provide immunizations and information about expectations for their age. Then, in the kindest manner, end the appointment by asking the inevitable: "Do you have any questions?"

Yea...about 35 million. Now what??? Is this it?! Is he too cold? Is he too hot? Where should she sleep? Am I doing this wrong? What's the best first food? Is he teething? Or is she sick? Do I need to give her that antibiotic? That shot? Is his latch right? Should I just pump? Give formula? What kind? How much? Why is she spitting up? Is that normal? Is he behind on his milestones? My friend's baby was rolling over by now—is something wrong with mine? He's still waking up like 6 times at night! I am non-functional —I don't know how much longer I can keep this up. I'm exhausted, scared, yearning for a shower, and on the brink of tears at any given point in the day. What do I do? Am I just supposed to power through? Is there another way?

Yes.

There is another way.

Does any of this sound familiar? Not only are these things I've heard countless patients say, but I've said them myself as well. The journey into parenthood is ROUGH! We only imagine the sleeping angels, and the sweet snuggles, and family photos. But real life is what happens in between those blissful snapshots. This process is hard, especially when you don't have a plan. A guide. Something or someone to support you in this journey. I never had one. That's not to say I didn't have support. I was lucky enough to have <u>tons</u> of family and friends willing to be there for me at the drop of a hat. But it doesn't matter when you're living in the postpartum world of mental fog and you can't even tell left from right or up from down. Love and support isn't the same as someone who's been through it all (maybe several times), and somehow made it out the other end. I know all I wanted in those early days was someone to empathize with me, yet simultaneously lead me judgement-free and walk with me on the journey in the direction I wanted to go.

This is the reason I chose to write this book. Between my 11 years in practice, seeing hundreds of women and their babies, and having my own 3 children, I have made ALL the mistakes myself, and I've seen nearly everything one can imagine that comes up when having a newborn-toddler stage child. Raising a healthy family is an incredible passion of mine. There are a lot of concepts that just aren't common knowledge that really should be! Information that should be conveyed in prenatal classes, but isn't. Facts about child rearing that offer choices, options, risks, and alternatives. But sadly none of this happens. Somehow, the concept that "it takes a village to raise a child," has faded away from our culture. Instead of being supported, we are constantly judged by peers on Facebook. The "mommy wars" have taken over our feeds, and as a result, new mothers feel oddly alone even when surrounded by loved ones. At a loss for answers even when "Dr. Google" is at our fingertips. Let's face it; "Dr. Google" is wrong more often than it is right. All it does is create anxiety over the worst case scenario. It's not worth it. There are other resources to get the insight you seek. But you have to know not only where to look, but what to ask. The bottom line is that I've felt the struggle firsthand and the desire to feel encouraged, supported, comforted, and reminded that we are not alone in this process.

I want to be that for you. You don't have to beat yourself up anymore. These aches and pains of motherhood are incredibly common, but they don't have to be "normal." We don't have to simply accept that these questions, heartaches, and states of confusion are just the normal state of affairs for the rest of your life. Or even the next year! You CAN reclaim your energy and clarity in your body and your mind! You CAN rekindle romance and connection with your partner again! You ARE enough for your baby and your family! And you WILL have the resources and support to know that you're making the right decisions for your child's well-being. There is a light at the end of the tunnel.

2

I've Been There

Mombie: A sleep deprived supermom who feeds on caffeine and survives on sticky kisses and smiles. Mombies are master multitaskers and suck-it-uppers.

I was a mombie. The first 1-2 years of my first child's life is literally a blur. I was young, newly graduated from chiropractic school, and truthfully wasn't expecting to get pregnant so soon. But, life happens! And we were ready for the ride. So we thought. I'd like to take this opportunity to share with you my story, and how I came out the other end.

My husband, Jason, and I had been married for almost 5 years when Evan was born in August 2010. That should have been sufficient time to have built a strong foundation of our relationship to withstand the stress a new baby brings to a marriage. It wasn't. We actually had started marital counseling about 3 weeks before finding out that I was pregnant. As soon as we knew, we were so elated that we discontinued therapy, feeling like this new bond of starting a family would magically fix whatever issues we previously had. But as my pregnancy progressed, my focus slowly and subtly shifted from only him and me, to baby and me. And while we were excited for the newness of pregnancy and the thrill of something out of the ordinary, we silently began more challenges. That said, my husband was amazingly supportive, and was at my side through every appointment and prenatal class. We took Bradley Childbirth classes to prepare for an intervention-free birth. I was grateful for this because, being a holistically minded physician, I wanted nothing more than a natural childbirth without induction/ pain medication. However, that didn't happen. It was a giant mess. A series of failures.

I was 9 days past my "due date." Yes— 9 days! I woke up at 7:15 a.m. feeling contractions! I was filled with excitement! *FINALLY, the time is here!!!* We took a walk, played card games, relaxed, and waited for labor to progress. By 5:00 p.m., I felt labor had gone on long enough and that we should head to the hospital. We arrived closer to 6:00 p.m., and my midwife proceeded to check me..."You're only 1 cm dilated. We cannot admit you until you're at 4 cm. We suggest you go back home and labor more and rest and come back when you're farther along. Seriously, you look too happy, and you still have makeup on. Go on home and come back later." Failure number 1.

So back home we went. Somewhere around 11:00 p.m., I began throwing up, and was feeling <u>miserable</u>. I was no longer "happy," and I'm pretty sure my makeup had been sweated off my face by now. At 1:00 a.m., we went back to the hospital, assuming SOMETHING must have moved forward.

"3 cm."

"You're welcome to stay in triage at this point for a few hours to see if you progress and then we can admit you instead of going all the way home again." Failure number 2.

So, in triage we stayed, with me pleasantly throwing up on and off for 4 hours. Peeing myself in the process. I was well beyond caring about my appearance. I no longer cared that I was falling asleep in between contractions on a hospital floor covered in my own urine. I just wanted to reach 4 cm so I could get into our natural birthing center room. Around 5:00 a.m., the midwife came in again. "It smells like amniotic fluid in here." *Is that supposed to be a compliment? WTF?!*

She checks me again, and woohoo!!! My water had broken (hence, the apparent smelling of amniotic fluid!) and I was at 5 cm! The birthing center room was occupied, but I was able to be admitted into a regular hospital room temporarily. *Thank God, at least now things are moving!*

But to my dismay, I stayed stuck at 5 cm for the next 20+ hours. I never moved to the ideal "birthing center" room. I got stuck in the "regular" hospital room. I received an IV to help with energy to encourage progression. No help. Failure number 3. They started me on Pitocin to speed up and intensify contractions. Failure number 4. By hour #40 of this process, I was done – physically, mentally, and emotionally. I was literally begging Jason to have them give me a C-section just to take this baby out. He had the presence of mind to know that my wishes were to have a vaginal birth. So, he talked me into simply succumbing to an epidural for pain control so that I could finally sleep after nearly 2 days.

Embracing my husband, I cried as I felt the needle go into my spine—but it was not due to the physical pain. It was from the pain of complete and utter exhaustion, and deep sadness. Failure number 5. My ultimate failure. My body let me down. My body let my baby down. Once I was able to appreciate the epidural for what it provided me—the elimination of pain and peace for the first time in nearly 2 days—I fell asleep. Three hours later, I was awakened by my midwife checking me, because my son's heartrate was triggering an alarm. My heart sank and I started to panic—*what now?!* I started crying again, thinking the worst. But thankfully, I learned that his heart rate was shifting as such, because I had finally reached 10 cm and was ready to push!!! Elated, I demanded that they discontinue the epidural drip so I could actually feel the contractions so as to push with functional muscles. An hour later, I had Evan in my arms, feeling relieved and grateful—but like a literal truck had run over me! I was beyond exhausted. In pain. Swollen from all the fluids. And now I had to look pleasant and smile for pictures as my parents and in-laws arrived to meet Evan and congratulate us. All the while I was in a complete daze, disconnected and dissociated from the trauma of the last few days.

As if my 5 perceived failures weren't enough, I was excited to exclusively breastfeed—but once again, life had other plans, apparently. Evan was still not back up to birth weight by a month old, and it was then that we discovered my severe lack of milk supply. Failure number 6. Not only did my body fail me in attempting to birth a child without interventions, but it wouldn't function enough to produce food to sustain his life and help him grow! He screamed all the time, which made sense if I was starving him. What a terrible mother I was turning out to be. I couldn't function. At the advice of my pediatrician, I kept him at the breast constantly. Performed skin to skin. Pumped. Swaddled him for comfort. But he was miserable. And so was I. I didn't recognize myself anymore, and I certainly didn't recognize this little creature that I was already a disaster in making. He finally got back up to birth weight by about 7 weeks of age, only after supplementing his feeds. Failure number 7.

So, my struggle with postpartum depression began. Although I literally didn't even know it until almost 2 years later! I lived those 20 months disconnected from Jason, Evan, and myself. Everyone was suffering—I sacrificed more and more, and had less and less. I didn't care about my birthday that year. I didn't care about holidays. This was starting the process of eliminating my own wants, needs, and myself from the equation of my life. Everyone I knew was supportive, and loved me, but couldn't see how unhappy I was. I can't blame them, as I didn't even realize what was going on. I even tried talking to a therapist about it at one point, as I was completely crushed at my birth experience happening the way it did. And my inability to breastfeed despite all my efforts and determination exacerbated my pain. I was laughed at. I was told, "You're upset because you needed an epidural? That's no big deal. And you can just feed formula, it's fine!" But it wasn't fine. My feelings and sadness were invalidated, and I sunk deeper into grief and felt like a failure. Even more so, because of my profession—it is my perspective that the innate ability of the body to heal itself is the greatest power on the planet. Everything can be achieved through natural methods. Sadly, it became apparent to me that my body and mind were the exception to that. It was also around that time that I learned my thyroid was underactive. Failure number 8-9? I lost count.

I also had this plan, this image, where I would be able to continue practicing at my office and just bring Evan with me while I treated patients. Being new in practice, I didn't have any staff or support available in my office. Just me, myself, and I. I had a pack and play in the corner of my treatment room, and I thought, "Perfect! I can just bring him with, and he can sleep in the pack and play while I work on my patients!"

You can guess how many times THAT happened! ZERO—he was fussy, needy, and never liked to be left alone. Over time, that took a grand toll on my energy, confidence, and self-worth. I began to only identify as "mama," and slowly lost other aspects of who I was as a person. I was left feeling so sad; while every smile and every milestone he made warmed my heart and soul to the very core, my life just wasn't the way I wanted it to be. The whole time, I just assumed this was normal motherhood. We become parents, and suddenly we no longer matter. Our needs are irrelevant and we just have to survive the next 18 years and then, and only then, we can potentially begin to find ourselves again, if it's possible by that point.

A series of things happened that allowed me to regain my own energy and my own power. It took a lot of time, and included a lot of care and treatments from colleagues of mine. Big thanks to Devon Acou, DC, and Cari Jacobson, DC, for their support on my journey! But I can tell you that it started with a decision. My decision. My choice that I no longer wanted to live in that fog. My decision to stop being a victim of my circumstances, and begin the steps of taking my life, my mind, and my body back. After weeks and months of consistent care, treatment, and many lifestyle changes and mental shifts, the cloud lifted and I was able to move on. But that was almost 2 years of Evan's life that I wasn't truly present for. And I can never get that time back. Luckily, I didn't make the same mistake again—when I had Noah 3 years later (I'll share his story in Chapter 6), I had much more energy, motivation, and mental clarity. It was thanks to all the steps and recommendations I will lay out in this book. Some may seem like common sense. Others are deeper. But either way, I wish that I had someone to show me this road map back then. Perhaps, if someone had, I wouldn't have had the experiences I did. However, all we can do is move forward. Then again, if I didn't have those experiences, it's likely that I wouldn't be here today sharing this book with you.

The bottom line is that I get it. I've felt all the shit and trauma, physically, mentally, and emotionally. Over the years, I've learned the process to overcome nearly anything. You don't need to feel depressed, exhausted, and like a giant mess. There is a healthier way to coordinate the chaos!

3

The Process

Don't just tell your children about the world. Show them.

Before we get started, I want you to know that this book is a judgement-free zone. We all make our own choices on raising our children, and that's ok. If everyone did everything the same way, the world would be boring and not be as diverse as it is! Different perspectives offer growth and opportunity. That's all I hope to provide you with here. An alternate perspective. Some new ideas. Or maybe some old ideas with a different spin. I want you to know that not everything we are told by our doctors, friends, family, and the media will work for everyone. And I want you to give yourself permission to do what feels right to you.

Repeat after me:

"It's ok to be different."

"It's ok to make mistakes."

"I get to make the decisions that I feel are best for me and my family."

That said, I know a lot of what you'll read in the coming chapters may come as a shock. Some things may sound intense, maybe even a bit crazy at first. Ride the wave. Hear me out. If you embrace a different path than what I present, that's ok! I'm not offended. You don't have to believe a thing I say—I simply invite you be open to some new things! Also, do your own research. Don't believe me—believe in yourself and your ability to read to find answers that resonate with you and your baby.

In the coming chapters, we will start with YOU. I want to make sure that you are centered and balanced, because let's face it —if mom is a mess, everything is a mess. This is why I start here. I help you understand specific ways to enhance your own energy through clear methods that you can begin today!

Next, we address your relationships. Your support systems. Your rocks. We've all heard it takes a village to raise a child. However, if that village fights constantly and is unhappy, then your child won't thrive growing up in that environment. And neither will YOU! This provides you the opportunity to truly evaluate your relationships to be sure they are supportive and positive in nature.

Last but not least, we get into each section of raising your new little person in this first year or so of their life. I'm here to assist and guide you on this road, but not dictate what path you take. You'll learn some new concepts and science behind my choices and I invite you to enjoy the process of learning. Please <u>don't</u> read anything and feel badly about yourself or your baby. We are only able to do the best we can with the resources and knowledge we have at the time. When we know better, we can do better. And my way is not always "better." Just different.

So, are you ready to jump in and start the journey of your healing and helping your child thrive?!

4

You! You Can't Pour From an Empty Cup

If mama ain't happy, ain't nobody happy!

This chapter may just be the most important part of this book. That quote is meant to be a joke, but there is a lot of truth to it. This entire process begins with our own healing. It starts with you being grounded and finding the deepest love for yourself, so that you can step into your own power. If you're miserable, unhappy and not thriving, you will NOT be able to be there for your child in the way that you want to be. YOU must come first in this scenario. It's the cliché lesson that we are taught every time we get on an airplane—"In the event that the cabin loses air pressure, and you're traveling with a child…." —who's oxygen mask do you apply first?! Your own. We as mothers have a tendency to be sacrificial lambs and put everyone else's needs before our own. That ends up serving no one, and makes us resentful and exhausted in the process. We are expected to give up EVERYTHING for our family. We give up our identity. We give up our romance. We give up our friendships. We give up fun and spontaneity. Sometimes, we even give up our careers when we have a child. Is this really necessary?! I'm here to inspire you to rethink that cultural conditioning.

I fell into that trap. It's so easy. As soon as that beautiful new little human came into my life, nothing else in my whole life mattered in that moment. I was in love, deeper than ever before. I was about to dedicate my life to making sure that I cared for him to the best of my abilities, and raised him to grow up to be an amazing human being. Prior to that moment, I never entertained the idea of being a stay-at-home mom. In fact, before having my first son, I actually looked down on women who gave up their careers to exclusively stay home. I used to think that it meant she didn't have a passion of her own to follow, or that it somehow made her weak to succumb to old-school gender stereotypes. But the second that I came home with my son, I got it. I totally understood the calling of that life. Every waking moment, I wanted to be there with him. To a new baby, mama is their everything. And it's what I wanted to be. At the same time, that's a lot of pressure. Yet, so many of us, out of instinct, reset all priorities upon becoming a parent. Most important is our child. Then a distant second is ourselves and our own needs, and last (if on the list at all) is our spouse or partner. Are you ready for my challenge?!

Put. Yourself. First. Period. This is not selfish. This is necessary. Now, I'm not suggesting that you become negligent and ignore the needs of your baby. Absolutely not. But if you're providing for his/her basic needs—they are fed, dry, warm, loved, and cared for—you have NOTHING to feel guilty about for taking a shower. You are not to shame yourself for wanting to get out of the house to exercise. Or to get coffee with a friend. Or even to go back to work. You were a human being before you created a new little one, AND you are a human being with needs and desires after, too. Under no circumstances should you deem it appropriate to put all your needs and wants on hold until after they have grown up. Because quite frankly, if you wait that long, it'll likely be too late to access who you truly are and reconnect with who you want to be. If we disregard the deepest part of ourselves for too long, it becomes incredibly difficult to get that back. Short term is one thing. If your child is sick, or in the early newborn stage, of course we are there for our children and we set aside our selfish desires for a few days/weeks/months until that stage has passed. But, it's time we start making self-care important. Because the bottom line is this: if you don't take care of yourself, you will have nothing left to give the people you care about. Burnout isn't sexy. It's not the goal. Yet, it happens every day to mothers around the world. We work our tails off to fill everyone else's metaphorical cup, that we forget to fill our own. When yours dries up, and you're empty? It's the most suffocating feeling on the planet. Tears can't begin to heal that pain.

So, how can we prevent that from happening? If you feel like you're already in that pattern, I promise there is hope. I'd like to introduce you to what I call the "7 best doctors" on Earth. They can and will help you get over anything. These are the doctors I want you to visit on a daily basis until your cup is filled to the brim and overflowing. Then, continue to fill it more! The overflow will simply fill more of your and your family's heart. These doctors I'm referring to are the following: 1) Sunlight, 2) Fresh Air, 3) Sleep, 4) Quality Diet, 5) Water, 6) Exercise, and 7) Joy. I'll go through each of these one by one to provide you details on how to take your life and vitality back, if you have neglected yourself and are experiencing that mama burnout.

SUNLIGHT

Get outside! The warmth of the sun will literally fill your soul. Sunlight by definition provides our soul literal and metaphorical light, and uplifts our mood without even trying. It will allow you a sense of peace, and create energy in your body. Obviously, sunlight is also necessary for the production of vitamin D! Vitamin D acts more like a hormone than it does a simple vitamin in your body. It has important roles in creating energy, establishing strong bones through calcium absorption, balancing stress hormones, supporting your immune system, and much more! Simply getting outside for some sunlight at least 20-30 minutes a day is critical for your health. The more skin you can expose to get the benefits of the vitamin D manufacturing, the better! Now, if you live in an area that doesn't have adequate weather or sunlight available all year round, then supplementation for D is necessary. Honestly, I believe sadly, that vitamin D supplementation is necessary for most of us, regardless of where we live. You can get a simple blood test to assess this now. I want your vitamin D levels to be at least 60-80ng/dl! So every day, regardless of the temperature, get outside for a few minutes. If the weather is nicer, make it at least 20-30 minutes per day. I understand the lack of desire to spend time outdoors when it's 14 degrees and snowing. Or, even worse, when it's 37 and rainy. So, in these scenarios, when you can't access the sun, this is where we can lean on vitamin D supplementation (or a safe indoor tanning bed) to get you through.

FRESH AIR

Just as I said above, nature is one of the most powerful energy aids we have at our disposal. Staying inside (as we've been forced to do through the 2020 Coronavirus pandemic), is NOT healthy. We all can feel a difference between breathing in the air from the inside of our homes, compared to inhaling deeply outdoors. I don't care how cold or warm it is—get outside and get grounded. I actually took a walk this winter outdoors twice weekly consistently as a friend and I talked on the phone, and it was one of the greatest things I did for my health! There were times the wind chill was -15, and I still bundled up and went out! It can be good for your baby, too! I know some cultures that have a regular practice of having their babies sleep outside while bundled up when it's below 30 degrees. This can actually be quite stimulating to their bodies and ours, offering a lot of benefits including reducing inflammation, increasing immune function, elevating mood, enhancing memory, and supporting mindfulness and peace. "Earthing" is a great practice too. This is where I recommend barefoot walking outside to access the unlimited potential of the earth's energy and electrical nature. This practice can fuel your energy and spirit and provide that sense of belonging and peace we all need.

SLEEP

This might be funny—you're the mother of a baby. You might be thinking—"Sleep?! What's that?!" I empathize, believe me. My kids didn't sleep through the night until they were WELL over 1 year old. And most nights, my 5-year-old still ends up in my bed. So, of all of these 7 doctors, this is the one I'll understand if you fall short. But try your best. I don't expect you to get 8 to 9 uninterrupted hours of sleep at this stage of your parenting time. But what you can do is focus on getting QUALITY sleep, if you're short on quantity. We've all heard the suggestions: sleep when the baby sleeps, laundry can wait, catch up on rest whenever you can! These recommendations, while well-intentioned, were not always realistic for me. If you're a napper, great—then nap! If not, don't force what's not there. If you're tired, sleep. Don't keep yourself up when you're tired as an attempt to have space when the house is quiet (at least not all the time!). Remember, sleep is a part of taking care of yourself. If you're too sleep deprived and a "mombie," your patience with your baby and your overall health will suffer. Sleep is where our bodies regenerate and heal. We as women are amazing as we are capable of functioning at this stage of life without a lot of sleep. But, just because we *can,* doesn't mean we *should.* Be mindful of your sleep goals. We actually will talk about this in more detail in a later chapter with regard to your baby's sleep!

QUALITY DIET

If you ask 10 people, you'll probably get 10 different answers on what qualifies as a "quality diet." But you're reading my book now, so you're going to get my opinion! ☺ Here's the secret: there is no "best" diet for everyone. However, I do believe there are some best practices that suit everyone regardless of your goals or opinions on nutrition. Eating real food is first and foremost what I recommend. As a new mother, I recognize the challenge of this. This means cooking your own food as opposed to picking something up that is precooked or prepackaged as a snack or meal. I have to tell you that your food supply is SOOOOOO important. Think about your car. Would you put diesel fuel in it if it was only designed for regular? Nope. Why not? Ask any mechanic and they'll tell you that it can ruin your engine, and if done enough without quick rectification, it can cause your vehicle to simply not run at all. Well, guess what? Your body is the most expensive vehicle you're ever going to own. It's irreplaceable. If you don't put the correct fuel in, over time you'll see the consequences. Garbage in = garbage out, as they say. This will manifest not only in how your body feels physically, but in how sharp, clear, focused, and stable we feel mentally and emotionally as well!

Let's start with the macronutrients. We need protein, fat, and carbohydrates. That's it. We don't need sugar. We're sweet enough! Carbohydrates frequently get a bad rap, but not all carbs are created equal. Remember that vegetables and fruits are carbs! Yes, so are bread, rice, pasta, potatoes, and cereals. The carbohydrates that come in whole food form are the best. Vegetables and fruits contain immeasurable benefits through the fiber, vitamins, minerals, and more! I can't say the same for the processed forms of carbohydrates. To create bread, pasta, cereals, etc. that we buy in the grocery store, all the nutrients are stripped away and fortified back in to provide shelf stability. This is why I always encourage a diet full of vegetables (organic, if possible) as a means to get your quota of carbohydrates in a day. Truthfully, we can get plenty of carbohydrates to meet our nutritional needs through vegetables only, and just a little bit of fruit. This is how I eat most of the time, minus an occasional birthday or holiday. I also highly suggest consuming twice as many vegetables each day than fruits. While fruit is nutritious, it *is* a sugar. Especially for those people who are sensitive to blood sugar spikes and drops, you may need to be mindful of which fruits are higher on the glycemic scale. (For example, banana, grapes, and melon tend to spike blood sugar more than the fruits in the berry family)!

Protein is next on my list of importance next to vegetables. I'm not a vegetarian, vegan, nor do I recommend most people adopt that lifestyle. There are healthy ways to keep a vegetarian or vegan diet, but it requires a lot of focus and dedication to keep the appropriate balance of protein to be sure you're not depleted in anything. Also, it's critical to supplement with vitamin B12 as it's primarily found in red meat. So, assuming you're not against eating animal foods, I like to highlight the importance and the difference in the quality of meats that we have the opportunity to purchase. I ALWAYS encourage buying grass-fed/organic animal products whenever possible. I promise the extra expense now is worth it. Eggs, beef, chicken—all should be grass-fed/organic. Fish should be wild-caught. Beans can be a good source of protein as well, but in limited quantities. I find that they can deplete your body of vital minerals when consumed too frequently due to their high levels of phytic acid.

Fats are the final macronutrient to discuss. I think this should go without saying now, but I need to be sure it's heard: FAT DOESN'T MAKE YOU FAT! Too much sugar and refined/processed carbohydrates will make you fat—and not only that, they cause diabetes, heart disease, high cholesterol, and inflammation that contribute to cancers and nearly all chronic disease. Fat is not to blame for these issues. However, there are good fats and bad fats. The fats I recommend consuming most are the following: avocado, extra virgin olive oil, organic butter, and coconut oil. Canola oil, vegetable oil, margarines, and trans fats of course are just plain toxic. When cooking at a high heat, my favorite oil to use is avocado oil as it has the highest smoke point, meaning that it will not denature and become free radicals in your body.

Olive oil should only be cooked with at a low to medium heat, or to drizzle on a salad. Below I've included a good resource to keep in mind for cooking oils healthfully, although note: I NEVER use Canola oil.

Oil	Smoke Point
Avocado Oil	520°F
Rice Bran Oil	490°F
Ghee (Clarified Butter)	450°F
Canola Oil	400°F
Grapeseed Oil	390°F
Lard	370°F
Butter	350°F
Coconut Oil	350°F
Extra Virgin Olive Oil	350°F

The bottom line when it comes to keeping and maintaining a healthy diet is this: Just eat REAL food! It's not as hard as it sounds, especially when you make it a priority and get used to it. In fact, Michael Pollan, acclaimed Amercian author and journalist, said something to the effect of this: Eat whatever you want!—Just make it yourself. Not only would the nutrients be higher in all food you make yourself, but how often would you eat certain things if you had to make them from scratch every time? Fries? Ice cream? Cookies? Pasta? We can focus on shopping the perimeter of the grocery store, and when we see anything from a package, scrutinize the ingredients to make sure the list is so simple you <u>could</u> make it yourself. We'll get more into this topic when we discuss feeding your baby in subsequent chapters, because I can tell you, it's much easier to get your child to eat healthy foods when you model the example! If you're looking for easy recipes, or more information to support my suggestions here, I would look up Paleo diet and/or Whole 30 on the Internet. There is a wealth of information out there if you know what to ask and what to look for!

WATER

I could write an entire book on the importance of water. When I see patients in my office, one of the most important things I address is their hydration status. I seriously find about 90% of people are somewhat dehydrated and don't even know it. Dehydration can lead to constipation, dry skin, and rashes, fatigue, mental fog, and more. Check out the book *Your Body's Many Cries for Water,* by F. Batmanghelidj, MD for more reasons to get hydrated! My formula for how much water to drink is simple: Half your body weight in ounces daily. So, if you're 150 lbs., you should drink 75 ounces of water each day. However, if you consume any caffeinated or alcoholic products, these beverages count as "negative" water because they act as a diuretic and deplete your body of hydration. Therefore, if you consume these items, you'll need to calculate that accordingly and add those "negative" ounces back in to get your ideal total water necessary to sustain your body optimally. So, in the above example, if you weigh 150 lbs., and you have 2 cups of coffee in the morning and 1 glass of wine at night, that's 20 additional ounces to add to your original amount of 75 ounces, totaling 95 ounces required.

Additionally, while I won't get into the details here, the kind of water also can make a big difference. I rarely recommend drinking tap water as your primary source. I find that one has to drink nearly twice as much tap water to compensate for the toxins and impurities present to achieve the same level of hydration. My favorite sources are spring, mineral, or high-quality filtered water like Berkey or Kangen. Brita filters do not remove enough, so unfortunately, they are not much better than tap water. It's one thing to drink some tap water when out to dinner, or from the drinking fountain at the gym from time to time. But generally speaking, 90% of the time, I suggest being mindful of the quality of water that you are consuming!

EXERCISE

Exercise is critical for so many reasons, the least of which at this point being cardiovascular health! For me, exercise was my "me" time. My release. My time away from the "mama" role. It gives me the opportunity, if only for a few hours a week, to simply move my body and feel free! Research has shown time and time again that regular, consistent exercise can be MORE effective at reducing depression and preventing anxiety than antidepressant medications. And this doesn't have to be fancy or intense workouts—simply walking for an hour, a few times a week can offer this effect. Now, I completely understand that especially early on in motherhood, you may not have the opportunity to sneak away to have this time to exercise alone. Do the best you can. Moving is better than not moving, but if it's possible, I HIGHLY recommend going for your walk or exercise alone. Taking the baby for a walk in the stroller, or your dog for a walk is great. But, if that baby starts to cry, or if your dog jumps off the leash or barks at another dog, that walk isn't about you. We all need our space, and I really want to encourage you from the mental health perspective to respect (and not judge) your need for it.

As far as what kind of exercise is right for you, more is not always better. It's really easy to overexert yourself to the point that exercising has the opposite effect of what's intended. I would almost always rather someone under-exercise than over-exercise. This concept will look different for everyone, of course. The appropriate amount and type of exercise is determined by your age, fitness level, and your particular goals. The way I recommend to keep track of your exertion level is through a simple heart rate monitor. The formula I use to calculate your ideal range is from Dr. Phil Maffetone, a physician and author of *Everyone is an Athlete*, and is the following: 180 minus your age, and then subtract 10 to get the range for your heart rate per minute. Example: if you're 30 years old, 180 - 30 = 150 - 10 =140. Therefore, your heart rate should be 140–150 beats per minute during exercise. This can be modified further depending on your fitness level and experience with exercising. If you're a seasoned athlete that has been working out at a high level for some time with no injuries, pain, or imbalances, then you can afford to push a little harder—up to 5–10 beats per minute higher. On the other hand, if you're recovering from an injury or trauma (AKA childbirth!!!), or other hormonal imbalances, it is likely best to reduce your exercise zone by 5–10 beats per minute. The point with this type of training is to meet your body where it is at so you can truly see your progress as your fitness level and efficiency improves. I actually trained for the Chicago Marathon this way (before having kids! ☺). By keeping a close eye on your heart rate, you monitor your intensity level while simply observing the work output. For me, this initially looked like a moderate walk. In September of 2008, I started consistently walking 5 times weekly at an approximate speed of 3.8 mph on the treadmill. Within a few months, I was walking more quickly. Within a few more months, I was alternating 4.5 mph jogs with 4.0 mph walking. And by the marathon in October 2009, my average speed running the entire thing was 5.3-5.5 mph! As I trained, I watched my heart rate remain constant and my ability to push harder and do more work increase! So, there is no shame in starting slow! I actually have to frequently teach my patients to start over in this way. And often they don't care for it. It can feel like you're not working out if you're accustomed to exercising too intensely. However, I can promise you it's worth it. Overtraining or exercising beyond the range I mentioned above consistently can hurt you in many ways:

- You're more vulnerable to injury
- You can create significant blood sugar imbalances
- You can deplete your body's energy, inducing chronic fatigue (which no new parent needs!)

These things can occur because exercising beyond your aerobic capacity or threshold puts enormous stress on your liver, adrenals, and pancreas. These systems work together to keep blood sugar balanced. Your adrenals in particular are responsible for all the stress in your life no matter where it comes from: emotionally, physically, thermally, chemically, electromagnetically, etc. While exercise should be a stress-reducer, overexertion quickly can make it a stress-creator. I've literally seen women in practice who eat really healthfully, have a happy balanced life, and yet they are anxious, in pain, and have blood sugar dysregulation or are on their way to diabetes simply due to exercising inappropriately.

Since I was about 19 or 20, I have had severe lower back pain at different points in life. Some years were better than others. During this time, I would seek chiropractic care on an as-needed basis. It was in my mid-thirties that it started getting worse than ever. I was running pretty consistently. Anywhere from 3-5 miles or more a day. At first the pain was slight, then month over month it got worse. I finally decided to follow my usual routine and seek out chiropractic care. But this time after months, it still wasn't getting better. The practitioner I was seeing at the time basically told me, if I continued to run, I was going to continue having back pain and further issues as I got older.

Speeding up, I met Dr. Christy about a year and a half ago. Shortly after, I made the choice to make the 2 ½ hour drive to consult with her. At the time I figured, "what is the worst thing that could happen at this point." And, I knew I already trusted her expertise. After my first visit I felt more relief than I did on any given visit at my previous practitioner. In the upcoming months, I learned a significant amount about how my adrenals and emotional wellness were playing a role in the pain. Dr. Christy helped heal my adrenals by teaching me how to exercise in the right zones, times, etc., and release the emotional factors associated with it. She also helped me better understand proper supplements and how even my water quality was playing a role.

Here we are now, nearly a year and a half later and other than the occasional flare up (which I can generally associate to pushing myself too hard in one way, shape, or form), the pain/discomfort I had in the past is nearly gone. And, I can finally run when I choose without the pain and discomfort simply by being better in tune to my body and what it needs.

Bottom line, often it's the basics that make the biggest impact! Thank you Doc!!!

-Jen Z.

JOY

Do you remember what joy is? And I'm not talking about happiness. Happiness, in my opinion, is a fleeting emotion that tends to be situationally dependent. Joy is a state of mind. It's part of who you are, regardless of your circumstances. For example, the coronavirus pandemic sucks! In fact, there are a lot of aspects of 2020 that were unfortunate, disappointing, and shitty to say the least. However, we have the power within us to be joyful anyway. What we focus on grows. Energy flows where we direct our attention. And I made the conscious, albeit sometimes difficult, decision to choose joy, gratitude, and love. Now, I know this is easier said than done. I encourage you to look for joy in everyday miracles: your baby's smile. A gentle breeze. Taking deep breaths. Keep a gratitude journal and remind yourself of all you have to be happy about. I also challenge you to find things in your life that provide you this sense of joy, peace, and love on a regular basis. Connecting with others, nature, meditation, art, journaling, photography, your career, exercise, or other hobbies....??? What are you passionate about? What makes your heart smile? What provides you energy and excitement? I'm personally passionate about health and my work. I get great fulfillment out of writing this book and developing content for my website, YouTube channel, and other social media. If I didn't have that, parenting would beat me into the ground. This is why it's more important now than ever for you to reflect deeply on who YOU want to be, and do what brings you that sense of joy. That looks different for everyone—there is NO WRONG ANSWER. ♥

Those 7 best doctors are simple. But I didn't say they were easy to follow on a regular basis. It's taken years of growth, work, and learning to get to a point where I can say I truly meet most of them consistently. Even today, though, I'm not perfect. No one is. I certainly don't expect someone who has a brand new little infant that is still healing from birth to achieve perfection! But what I can tell you is that the awareness of the ultimate goal of what you want is the first step in healing and balancing your body and your life. I was a guest on a podcast in February 2021 entitled *Finding Your Village,* and the host, Amanda Gorman, shared something brilliant on this topic. She suggested making a list of all the things that you can do to fill your cup. Reference the above "doctors" and list all ways that would best make you feel peaceful, stabilized, and happy. Because when we have a few minutes or just maybe a few hours when the baby is asleep, the last thing on our mind is self-care. But if you have things written down that you can easily reference when tired or distracted, it will help refocus your attention on yourself, and provide you some options for what to do with your precious time! Anything that we can do to keep our own health and joy top of mind is critical. Furthermore, let's not underestimate the power of miniature versions of self-care that you can embrace daily: a 5-minute, uninterrupted shower, closing the door when going to the bathroom, peeing when you need to and not holding it for an hour, a minute outside alone for a breath of fresh air, some deep breaths before getting up to start your day. I'd argue those aren't "self-care," but increasing the awareness of these little things is better than nothing!

Before we get to hormones, I want to address one more thing: ENERGY. This is sometimes a difficult topic to understand, but follow me here. What color did you paint your baby's room?

Pastels? Neutral? Pink? Blue?

Did you paint it black?

Why not? Because that wouldn't *feel* right. Painting an entire room black would not have the right energy for your child to thrive, and sleep well, right? Energy is this annoyingly intangible thing that everyone can feel but no one can explain. We as a human race feed off one another's energy all the time—and our kids do so even more due to the bond we share with them as mothers. We are the example for our kids on EVERYTHING. How we eat, dress, think, speak, act in relationships—this list can go on. That's of course a lot of pressure on us. But the bottom line is to be sure that our own cup is full. When we are drained, there is nothing for us to give, and literally EVERYONE suffers as a result. And what is one of the best ways to reset your energy, in all senses of the word?

MEDITATION

Meditation sometimes freaks people out. Many assume there is a specific way to do it correctly, and if you're not doing it "right," it won't have the desired effect. This couldn't be farther from the truth. The only "wrong" way to meditate is to not do so at all. The goal of a meditation is to calm your mind, become centered in the present moment, and simply breathe and connect within. There are literally dozens of ways to achieve a meditative state to gain this balance and groundedness that we all seek. The focus is to choose something that will enhance that calm within your mind and body—my only rule is that watching a show or scrolling on your phone isn't meditative. It can absolutely put you in a trance, but those devices/screens suck you in and don't allow for that present moment grounding experience. Instead they create a dependency and a sense of being unsettled, which is the opposite of the goal. Here's a handful of ways that I recommend my patients get started if they're stumped on the best way to meditate:

BREATHING/FORMAL MEDITATIONS

Simply sitting still focusing on your breath is a simple and powerful way to meditate. When doing this, I want you to work on diaphragmatic breathing—allow yourself to take deep, slow breaths in and out, feeling your abdomen expand and relax with every breath. There are many apps available now to help guide you through this process to keep you on track. I'll include some resources for this at the end of the book. I know my mind tends to wander easily to my "to do" list when trying to settle. This is NORMAL—it doesn't mean you're failing or suck at meditation. It means you need to do it more! My rule of thumb is to give yourself 5 minutes each day to reset your mind and body through a form of meditation. And if you can't make time for 5 minutes per day, you need to do 10! ☺

JOURNALING

Writing your thoughts, fears, and aspirations has power. Keeping limiting belief patterns in your head doesn't allow them to escape. Just as keeping empowering thoughts inside doesn't serve you. Get these stressors and exciting ideas out of your head and onto some paper. It is frequently cathartic to physically get this emotional release through journaling. How you address these entries will vary depending on your particular life stressors. Issues with a particular person? Write them a letter. (You do NOT have to send it!). Write yourself a letter. Writing with the intention of talking to someone specific will change the energy of your tone and context, providing it more power. After you're done, what you do with these is your decision. Burn it? Save it? Share it? It's completely your decision to determine what will ultimately give you the most peace and satisfaction within.

COLORING/PAINTING/ART

I'm sure you've seen these adult coloring books. Personally, I'd prefer coloring my kid's coloring pages of dinosaurs and animals. The adult coloring pages with the complex array of lines and micro spaces to color causes me more stress. But, especially if you like art, coloring has been shown in studies to reduce physiological stress as much as a formal meditation—once again proving my point that there is no wrong way to do this! If you're an artistic person, paint! Draw! Sketch! Let the creative juices flow naturally, and you'll likely enjoy where they lead you and how you feel afterwards!

WALKING

If you're a more physical person, don't discount the power of moving your body for release. I hear frequently from patients that they take their dog for a walk every day, or push the stroller to get out with the baby, or take evening strolls with their spouse every night. These are all great, but assuming it's safe and possible to do so, I implore you to go alone. As I said before, if you want this to be "you" time, going for a walk alone has incredible healing power. It doesn't have to be long—a meditation walk is not the same as a walk/run intended for exercise. That said, exercise can absolutely provide this too. I'm just encouraging you to set aside extra time for this.

Ok, time for hormonal talk!

Let me start off by saying that we have a problem in our society—we have a tendency to equate what is "common," for what is considered "normal." Just because headaches are common, doesn't mean they are normal. Just because painful periods are common, doesn't mean they are normal. In the same way, just because postpartum depression, anxiety, hair loss, and overwhelming stress are common in parenthood, doesn't mean it needs to be accepted as normal. Hormones absolutely play a large role in all of the above, and the healthier a woman is, the more balanced her hormones are. That said, for several months postpartum, it is relatively normal *and* common for your hormones to be all over the map. What we need during that time is mental, emotional, nutritional, and physical support to stabilize them. The "7 best doctors" that I discussed first completely influence your hormone's release, function, and balance throughout your body. So, first and foremost, address those simple yet profound concepts, or you may as well not bother working on your hormones. I know that the harder I work on keeping the basics of my health in check, the less specialized work I need to do in other areas of my physiology.

My first recommendation to begin stabilizing your hormones is to find a holistic/functional medicine physician that can work with your specific body to determine its needs.

Check your thyroid. Check for antibodies too, as sadly it is all too common these days to slip into an autoimmune thyroid state postpartum. (I did!) Your Thyroid Stimulating Hormone (TSH) level should be between 1 and 2. If it's between 2 and 3, your doctor may think it's fine and normal, but it's not optimal. A functional/holistic physician can help navigate you through the process of determining appropriate levels for you. Here is the list of lab tests I would recommend getting when you have the opportunity:

TSH, Free T3, Free T4, Anti-TPO antibodies, Anti-Thyroglobulin antibodies, Reverse T3, Cortisol, Prolactin, Testosterone, Estrogen, Progesterone, HbA1C, Comprehensive Metabolic Profile (CMP), Complete Blood Count (CBC w/ diff), and Lipid Panel.

Depending on your age and amount of months postpartum, there will be different recommendations, which is why I'm not writing all ideal ranges here. After determining your ideal, supplementation may be required, but once you find the right combination of minerals/vitamins/herbs, you'll feel that cloud lift and have the clarity you seek.

For me, I needed thyroid support. For someone else, it may be best to focus on stabilizing blood sugar. For others, the priority may be herbs to balance all the hormones. Everything here is so personalized and different for everyone. If you're experiencing any of the typically "normal" postpartum symptoms, investigating further is critical. Like I shared with you in Chapter 2, I feel a lot of sadness for who I was and the state that my mind and body were in after the birth of my first son. Thankfully, I did a lot of work on myself to become a lot more energetic and balanced with #2 and subsequently #3!

Something I'd like to introduce you to if you're not aware of it already is called placenta encapsulation. It may sound gross, and it's absolutely not for everyone, but when used appropriately, it can be VERY effective in supporting you in the first month or so after having a baby. Essentially, this involves having a postpartum doula take your placenta after birth, sterilizing it, freeze drying it, blending it and placing the dried powdered remains into capsules for your consumption. Sometimes it's infused with herbs, other times not. Once again, this is dependent on your needs. Obviously I didn't do this after I had Evan—I wasn't aware of it as an option. I chose to encapsulate my placenta with Noah, my 2nd born, and it was a HUGE GAME CHANGER! I was energized. I was mentally clear. I was happy. I felt grounded. Now, I'm sure some of it was not being a complete novice to the whole parenting thing. But I can guarantee you that those little pills made a big difference for me. I feel it even helped support my milk supply a bit. I did it after having my 3rd son as well, and while it helped, I could tell that my body was in a very different place, and it wasn't as effective or necessary for me at that time. I'll explain why this is true a bit more in Chapter 6 where we discuss the significance and impact your birth experience can have on your body and on your baby.

Lastly, the other thing that I encourage you to look into when looking into practitioners to help support you on this journey is a system called Neuro-Emotional Technique (NET). At the end of the book, I'll have an entire section of resources for you, including where you can go to find the right healers. NET is a system that helps disconnect the stress from your past and subconscious beliefs from your body. Stress is a constant in our lives, and while we can't change the stress that's present, there are certain modalities and therapies that can stop the stress from impacting your body negatively. These types of modalities also support a reframe of those perspectives that may be disempowering to you and your life. I personally use NET in my practice, and have had it utilized on me when trying to break through old patterns and limiting belief systems. This system, as many that I use, involves muscle testing, and tapping into the energy of your body, correlating weaknesses with emotions and their corresponding organ system or meridian imbalances. We can then take this information and essentially, through muscle testing, access the details as to where and when the triggering event or events began. When identifying these patterns, we then clear the nervous system of the hold that those emotions have on your cells in your body. It's incredibly powerful!

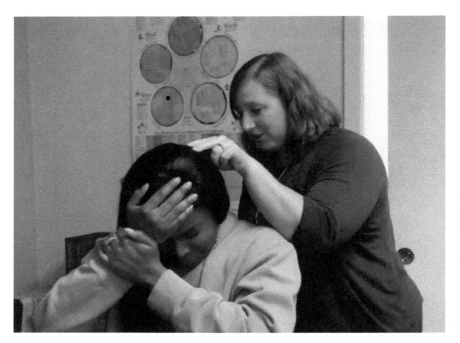

An example of my utilizing NET with a patient

Here's an example of how this works. When I start working with a patient, of course I take a detailed history and do a thorough examination. Once we start treatment, there are various reflexes on the body that correspond to different organs, as well as other imbalances such as emotional distress, illnesses, and more. When someone tests weak to an emotional reflex, this opens the door to begin utilizing this technique. We narrow down by asking the person and testing their muscles simultaneously for the primary issue "you?" "money?" "love?" Those are the most common categories, although, of course we can find more. Once the major category of stress is identified, I determine through muscle testing which organ/correlating emotion is indicated. These are the primary emotions that relate to each organ system/meridian. This chart is very important, as when we aren't fully reflecting on, and processing our emotions, those patterns can get stuck and literally cause physical problems in the area they primarily effect. (The reason there are two organs listed on each line is due to the element in which they belong and are paired with in Chinese Medicine—Wood, Metal, Earth, Fire, Water).

Liver/Gallbladder – Anger, resentment, frustration…
Lungs/Large Intestine – Defensiveness, stuck, grief, sadness…
Stomach/Spleen-Pancreas – Worry, over-concern, low self-esteem…
Thyroid/Adrenals – Unsure, paranoia, emotional instability…
Small Intestine/Heart – Lost, vulnerable, insecurity…
Kidney/Bladder – Fear, dread, paralyzed will…

After our muscle testing narrows the focus of what meridian and emotion are being triggered, the patient then reflects on how they connect that emotion with the concept of what came up (love, money… etc.?). Once again, to uncover the root of the issue, we then take it back further to the original event and narrow down an age or approximate age in which the root belief or issue was developed. As in the picture, the patient then places their hands over the emotional reflexes in the forehead, while I tap various spinal levels that accompany the organ/meridian in question. The patient deeply breathes and lets go of that original event, breaking the connection so it no longer has a physical or neurological impact on their body. Personally, as a mom, this system has been so beneficial to me! Patients report feeling lighter, more energized, grounded, and clear after NET sessions. What mom doesn't need that!? ☺

The take home message of this chapter is to TAKE CARE OF YOURSELF!!! Self-care has never been more important than it is now, and ironically, this is the time of your life that it begins taking a back seat. Love yourself and your family enough to fill your cup first. Physically, chemically, and emotionally—anything in your world can affect anything in your body. Spend the time and take the care to reflect on your health frequently. By checking in with yourself and making the 7 doctors, your hormonal balance, and emotional health a priority, most stress in your external world will be much more manageable! As we go through the rest of the important steps in getting your humanity back and helping your kids thrive, never forget the most important person in this process: YOU.

5

Your Relationship

Happily ever after is not a fairy tale. It's a choice.
-Fawn Weaver

Part two of this process, second only to working on yourself and your own needs, is to focus on your relationship. Now, for the purposes of this chapter, I'm going to be primarily referring to your romantic partnership. I will use terms like "husband," "spouse," and "partner." I will use these terms interchangeably, but under no circumstances am I judging the status of any relationship. Please take this content and apply it to your situation. I do not care what your family dynamic looks like, as long as it's healthy and fulfilling to you. Homosexual or heterosexual relationships, marital partnerships, simply living together, single/co-parenting—these labels do not matter. Additionally, if you are divorced or separated from the partner with whom you had a child, this does not mean this chapter doesn't apply to you. In fact, you un-derstand more than ever how important this piece of the puzzle is. If you're not currently in a romantic relationship, you can extrapolate the recommendations here towards any relationship that is important to you and the well-being of your child. My goal with this chapter is to get you evaluating your important relationships that are going to be your and your baby's primary support systems. If you're a single parent, please consider your closest friends, parents, significant other,

other family or siblings to be sure that you nurture those relationships similarly as described here for the deepest impact. Remember, we discussed last chapter the importance of putting yourself first—if you're depleted, there is nothing left to provide others. The same goes for your partner—if you neglect him/her, your connection with them becomes depleted quickly, weakening you as a unit. A child can place an enormous strain on a relationship. If it wasn't strong before, it can easily break if not attended to and nurtured.

I'm going to introduce a concept here that you may already be familiar with. If you are, it's worth repeating. If not, this is critical information to encouraging the development and deepening of your intimate relationship. My husband and I recently read a book together that drastically shifted the awareness we each had of each other, and strengthened our connection. That book was written by Dr. Gary Chapman, and entitled *The 5 Love Languages.* In the book, he makes the point that each of us show/receive love differently. Love is a language, just like any other—Spanish, French, English, etc. If you're speaking a language that is different than your partner, the message sent will not be the message received and challenges will arise as a result. And not always, of course, but *usually*, the way one expresses love most frequently is the way they prefer to receive it. The language we speak is generally the language we comprehend best. Just like we discussed in the last chapter, commonly the first step to healing your relationship is first to look within, reflect on yourself and apply that knowledge to your partnership. I highly recommend reading this book. I've known about the 5 love languages for some time, but was dead wrong in my assumption about what my primary language was. It was upon actually reading the book and taking the quiz that I discovered my deepest love language, which I spoke when letting go of all external expectations. It's a very quick read, but if you don't have the time, at least check out the quizzes and information at https://www.5lovelanguages.com/.

So, let's go through these one by one.

WORDS OF AFFIRMATION

Words of affirmation can be as simple as telling your spouse, "I love you." "I'm proud of you." "I appreciate you." It can also be as intricate as a love letter, a hand-written poem, acknowledgement on their looks after a new haircut or outfit purchase, or inspirational quotes provided for him/her. The important part here—when your partner's love language is words, written or verbal, your communication carries energy and power with them. Your partner needs to *hear* that you love, care, appreciate, and are grateful for them regularly. Otherwise, their take-home message is that they are not loved.

ACTS OF SERVICE

Acts of service are specific things one does for their partner. Often times these actions are chores, but they don't have to be. Cooking, cleaning, and laundry are some obvious ways to support someone when their primary love language is acts of service. However, what can be just as cup-filling, so to speak, can be washing your spouse's car, or doing the grocery shopping when it's not usually your role. Doing a surprise for the other goes a long way too!

QUALITY TIME

Quality time probably feels like one of the most challenging ones to accomplish during this time of your life. At this point you eat, sleep, breathe baby, and there's very little time for anything else. However, if you ignore your relationship for too long, before long you'll notice the disconnection and the difficulty in healing it. If your partner's language is quality time, all they want is TIME together. Uninterrupted, undistracted, focused love. So, date nights (or more likely date minutes or hours) are a must if this is your/your partner's love language. Just simply being together in the same space can be enough for some to fill their spiritual cup of connection with you.

RECEIVING GIFTS

Receiving gifts may seem obvious. This is where a person prefers to actually receive a present from their spouse as their way of feeling loved, cared for, and appreciated. The sneaky thing is that many things can qualify as a "gift" to those with this as their love language. Simply one's presence can qualify, a note, flowers, etc. Most of the time, gifts do not need to be monetary or expensive. Creativity can go a long way, and the meaning behind it is most important.

PHYSICAL TOUCH

Physical touch does not necessarily mean sex. Of course, it is one way of physically being intimate, and to those with a primarily touch love language, sexual intimacy is much more than just physical. It's truly one of their ways of connecting and experiencing love. However, nonsexual touch can be just as effective at supporting your partner's touch tank. Hugs, holding hands, snuggling to a movie, a back massage, foot rub, or a simple kiss are some other affectionate ways to satisfy a need for physical touch. Just ask your spouse what their preferences are.

The bottom line with any love language is that what we focus on and put energy towards will grow. If we focus on the energy drain, fatigue, disconnection, lack of intimacy, and decreased support, then we will get less of our needs met and our relationship will become further challenged. This is why I said in the last chapter—our children are very important, but they are not the only important thing in our lives. We need to come first. If our cup isn't full, there is nothing left for us to give our family. Similarly speaking, if we fail to nurture our relationship in the way that our partner recognizes, a divide will slowly form—and before you know it, 10 years will pass by and you won't know where to begin to repair it.

This is what happened to my husband and me. We don't speak the same love language. My primary languages are receiving gifts/acts of service/words of affirmation, and his are physical touch/quality time. This was not something we came to recognize until recently. We were married nearly 15 years before opening our eyes. Little things stood in our way of meeting each other's needs, and I sabotaged my own love language for years. When money was tight, I specifically told him not to buy me anything for my birthday, Christmas, our anniversary, Valentine's Day or any other holiday. I decided that wasn't important. I put myself last. At the time I thought quality time was most important to me. (It was in reading the book last year that I realized it was his presence that represented a gift to me). Things slowly started to break down between us even before my first son was born. But it got worse once I became a mother.

I had a lot of subconscious expectations of myself upon becoming a parent. I absolutely fell into the trap that my life was no longer mine to live. My spouse was no longer my partner, but the father of my child(ren). We gradually began relating to each other only as parents instead of husband and wife. An added stressor was the fact that as a new mother attempting to breastfeed, I was "touched out" constantly. Not great when your husband's love language is physical touch. So, between me directly sabotaging what would have been any attempt to meet my love language, and me not having any interest in his, the divide grew insidiously. Things would stabilize a little bit as each child grew older and would easily slip back after another pregnancy and baby. Hence, why I'm preaching this now! If you don't make your relationship a priority at this moment, it may be too late when you think you "have time."

That's the thing about "having time" for people or things. I don't "have" any more time than anyone else. We are all gifted 24 hours each day to do with what we will. We allocate our hours to what is our priority. I don't "have" time to workout—I "make" time to workout at least 4 times per week because it's important to me. I don't "have" time to cook healthy meals for my family, but I "make" the time because it's my priority. And I don't "have" time to cultivate a deeper bond with my husband, but we are MAKING the time, because we know the alternative is living unhappily and disconnected. This is a hard pill to swallow sometimes—and SOMETIMES, time really does get in the way—but the truth is, the majority of the time, what you "don't have time" for just isn't that important to you. My phone reminds me constantly about how much screen time I use on an average day. If I weren't addicted to my phone, how much more time could I dedicate to other areas of my life?!

Now here's the thing, some relationships may not be meant to be. That is for you to determine. I could cite all the studies and information to tell you that a 2-parent household is better in many ways for a baby's development, security, and many levels of stability (mental, emotional, financial, academic, etc.). It is not new information that a child growing up in a stable 2-parent home is ideal. However, it does the child NO good to grow up in an environment where his/her parents aren't happy. Not only does the energy and dynamic of your relationship affect the energy of the child and home, your interactions with your spouse set an example for what a relationship should be. It may not seem significant now, but as your baby grows, they look to you for what's acceptable in a partnership. I'm absolutely an advocate of working on it under most circumstances. But not all. And if there is abuse going on, whether verbal or physical, there is no fixing that, and I recommend getting out and seeking support and help immediately! For those relationships where there is no abuse, and life has simply gotten in the way of who you both used to be, WORK ON IT. Romantic relationships aren't always easy, and I have a handful of tricks that I've read and used personally to begin the process of rekindling that flame.

How did you meet? What first attracted you to one another? What were some fun things you enjoyed doing together before marriage/baby? Before kids? My husband and I used to enjoy mini golf, bowling, outdoor activities, concerts, and fun! Guess what went out the window when we became parents? All of that! Now, it's obvious that a lot of those kinds of activities will be limited once a small human comes into your life (or when a pandemic is upon us!). But just because it doesn't occur as often as it did when you were dating doesn't mean it shouldn't happen at all. Sometimes we need to get creative. Bonding with your spouse is not an all or nothing kind of thing. I encourage you to make a list of things with your partner that you both enjoy(ed) doing before your baby was born. Then see what you can still make happen from time to time! Even if it's only a monthly (or less frequent sometimes) date night!

Now, let's talk about date nights. They are everyone's advice right? Get together and there's one cardinal rule: Don't talk about the baby! First of all, that is ridiculous. I understand the sentiment behind that suggestion, but I think it's completely unrealistic. This new person in your life is a huge deal, and it's totally normal to want to talk about the baby with the person who helped create him/her! There's no reason to expect you to shut off that part of your heart. Now, that said, your baby shouldn't be the ONLY thing you discuss when on a night out. But if he or she comes up a few times, that's ok and shouldn't be condemned or feel "taboo." Secondly, what if finances are a struggle? Or you don't live near family that can babysit frequently to support these date nights? It's a great idea in theory, but we need to find ways to connect over the ordinary. The boring. The monotonous. The day-to-day. Make that decision and smile, and create that sense of joy in your body, and it will drive you to love your spouse like you did when you first met. My husband and I created a weekly date night "in," after the kids went to bed where we would do something together for a few hours. Something that encouraged communication and fun.

What if you're already there? I have several patients in their 50s that are about to be "empty nesters," and the women feel empty, disconnected, and estranged from their husband of 20+ years. Divorce is on the table, but not even easy to pursue after that much time. All they know is that they are unhappy, and they don't want to live the next 40 years that way. There is a way to avoid becoming this. IT TAKES EFFORT. Reread that part about making your spouse a priority. If we don't make time for our relationship, we'll end up making time for our divorce. So, if you're already feeling like you're headed down that path, I'll share with you a few things that have helped us get past that point.

Up until now, we really didn't ever have much therapy or marital counseling. We were never opposed to it—in fact we pursued it for awhile but decided against it for financial reasons. But just because we didn't get professional help doesn't mean we sat on our asses and did nothing. We read the aforementioned *Love Languages* book together. We discussed every chapter, took notes, and shared insights and thoughts. When that was done, we found a new book to read together with which to learn about our relationship and grow closer. We read a chapter a week and once weekly we would convene to exchange thoughts and our planned work to do. Consider it like our own version of therapy! Lastly, ask each other questions! A friend bought us a book of questions that are meant to spark conversation among couples. Some questions are simplistic, others provoke deeper reflection. We actually used to do this when out to dinner in our early periods of parenthood. We'd come up with hypothetical questions to get us talking about something other than the kids. What would we do with the money if we won the lottery? Where are our top 5 vacation spots? What are our personal/couple/family goals for the coming year? This type of conversation begins the process of connecting again, and we all need it. I'll be honest, my husband and I are not yet where I'd like to be as far as connectedness and relationship stability is concerned. We have more than our share of issues that we are working on. But we are

ACTIVELY working on them. "Nothing changes if nothing changes." -Courtney C. Stevens.

This entire chapter is about the deep importance of one word: connection. There are many ways to connect with your partner, and all are equally important: physically, spiritually, sexually, and emotionally. What I described above with the books and questions are great for engaging spiritual and mental/emotional connection. Just like the love languages, we all generally have differing levels of needs for each, but we can't neglect the aspects of nurturing the relationship just because they may not be our primary focus. It may feel awkward to talk about—but let's talk about SEX!

In my experience, (and experiences shared with me from many men and women over the years), women need to feel connected emotionally with their spouse before they are capable of wanting to connect sexually. For men? It's the opposite. They need to connect sexually first before they feel comfortable and willing to open up to connecting emotionally. So how does either party get their needs for love and connection met? Compromise. Connection feeds more connection. And disconnection feeds more disconnection. So, pick one and start. Once you get into a new pattern that's less destructive, you'll be well on your way to rekindling the spark you once had. Libido is a different story and can be related to hormonal imbalances discussed in the last chapter. If all hormonal issues have been ruled out by a functional medicine specialist, then the only thing you're left with being the issue is lack of interest in your partner. No matter how you think of it, sex is critically important to a marriage. Sex is the defining difference between a romantic relationship and a platonic friendship. Friendships are grand! I'm lucky to have several close friends to whom I can turn anytime! My spouse is a different level of a friend. He knows me like no one else. He has seen me through the worst and then some. I've also likely treated him the worst. We tend to treat those we are closest to the worst as we are most comfortable with them, and feel the most trust.

It's ass-backwards, but true. What if we created a new pattern? Rewrote this story? The power is within us to create the relationship we want.

We <u>need</u> fun in our lives, and humans are social beings. It wouldn't be natural for us to raise our young in a cave, disconnected from our partner. That may be the norm for other species in the animal kingdom, but human beings require intellectual stimulation, growth, and connection to thrive. To what degree of each is dependent upon the person and the couple. So, talk about it with your partner! Ask each other about your goals, passions, dreams, and how to have more fun! When I mentioned expectations earlier, my subconscious one was that I was no longer able to have fun as a mother—I'm sorry for my language here, but WHAT THE FUCK?! I look back at that BS belief ("BS" actually stands for "belief system" AND "bull-shit" as they are usually synonymous)! It's time to consider your goals for your relationship, your family, and your life. Remember, it may sound cliché, but our lives are meant to be abundant in all areas. Just because it's not what we see on a regular basis, doesn't mean it's not possible or worth going after. I suggest also maybe finding a couple that could potentially mentor you—someone you respect and see their joy, love, passion, and effort that is in their relationship. We look up to celebrities and employers in differing contexts; partnerships can be the same way. It's time to have fun and create what you want, starting now. ☺

6

Baby's Birth Significance

"Birth matters, and I believe the way a child is brought into the world has an important impact on the rest of life."
-Anjli Aurora Hinman, CNM

What was your baby's birth like? As I shared with you earlier, my experience in my birth story with Evan was completely devastating to me. It literally took me years to get past the trauma and grief that I felt. And there's one point that I want to drive home here: <u>it's ok to grieve your birth experience.</u>

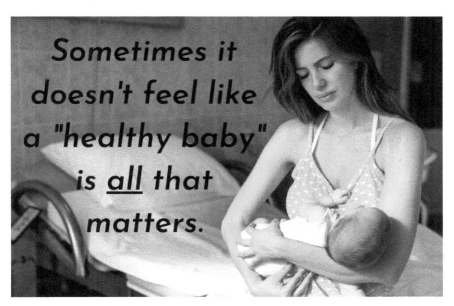

Sometimes it doesn't feel like a "healthy baby" is <u>all</u> that matters.

After we have our first child, all our well-intentioned family members and support team of doctors and nurses, tell us the same thing: "All that matters is that you and the baby are healthy." And they are absolutely right—I'm so very thankful that I never had any bigger health issues myself or with my babies. My heart breaks for those families who have had their lives shattered from infant loss or other traumas/injuries/anomalies. I know many women with stories like this, and the grief and deep sense of emptiness never truly leaves. It changes with time, but it is always there. Regardless of your individual birth story sequence of events, birth is an incredibly personal experience. Each woman connects with the process differently. I know plenty of women who had to have a C-section delivery after hours of attempting a vaginal birth. Many come out of that experience with the perspective that their body failed them or that somehow they were less of a woman/mother as a result. This can frequently lead to the interpretation of birth trauma and grieving the loss of an intended "birth plan." I thank God that those sorts of medical interventions exist for true emergencies. The problem is, in my opinion, induction, augmentation of labor, epidurals and C-sections are not as necessary as frequently as they are routinely performed. These interventions do not come without risk.

Birth is a normal, natural process! The female body was intended for this. It's not as scary as many doctors make it out to be. Now, don't get me wrong—labor and delivery SUCKS. I'm not going to bullshit you and say that it's a pleasant experience. I had 3 very different types of birth experiences—I'd like to share the other 2 with you now. Through this narrative, I want to illustrate the difference in my own mental state, energy, recovery, and my child's disposition as it related to each birth.

I already shared Evan's story with you. So, when I was pregnant with our 2nd, I was bound and determined to have a different experience than the first time around. I got a lot of regular chiropractic care, and energetic/emotional balancing work to help me work through the pain from Evan's birth. I also had a brief hypnotherapy session with a colleague at my office the day before beginning my maternity leave (10/16/13). So, it was Thursday morning October 17, 2013. I went to my midwife's office for my routine appointment. Being 8 days late, I had a non-stress test and ultrasound to assess that everything was still healthy. Things were fine, so I asked my midwife to check me. At 12:30 p.m., I was already dilated 2.5 cm and 80% effaced. As I was ready to get the party started, I had Brigitte sweep my membranes that day. She warned that I may feel some mild cramping as a response to the sweep and that it may/may not turn into labor. She was right. To be honest, I can't say when labor officially started. It could've been as early as 3:30 p.m. when I was finishing treating my last patients beginning my maternity leave. It could've been 6:00 p.m. as we were eating dinner, or 9:00 p.m. before going to bed—either way, the onset of "official" early labor is vague. I was pretty certain before going to bed that night that it was starting, so for all intents and purposes, let's call it 9:00 p.m. 10/17 = onset of early labor. Mild cramping every 3-5 minutes lasting 30-60 seconds. So, I went to bed. I woke at 1:00 a.m., still in labor. Peed. Back to bed. I woke at 3:00 a.m., still in labor. Peed. Back to bed. At some point between 3:00 a.m. and 5:00 a.m., Jason gets awakened by my grunting through contractions in my sleep and realizes that I'm in labor. At 5:00 a.m., I woke again. Peed, and I slept on/off between contractions until 7:00 a.m. Here's where it gets interesting. Below is the list of things we VOWED to do differently, having had the past experience we did:

- ✓ Stay home AS LONG AS POSSIBLE!
- ✓ Sleep more!
- ✓ Drink more water!
- ✓ Eat more for energy!
- ✓ Walk more to enlist gravity's assistance in progressing things!

We were working on our list, and doing well. By 7:00 a.m. contractions were about 3 minutes apart, lasting about 1 minute and 15 seconds each. They sucked, but were bearable. Jason was getting Evan situated with my parents, making breakfast, getting car packed, and coaching/massaging me as needed. We talk to our midwife at 8:00 a.m., and she essentially tells us that we can leave for the hospital anytime. So by about 8:35 a.m., Jason tells me that everything is ready and it's time to go. I was on the brink of my next contraction, so I wanted to stay for that one before having to walk out to the car. I get through it, roll over, and BAM!!! My water breaks. I stand up, knowing now we REALLY need to go. Halfway to the door, I collapse on my hands and knees with the urge to push. (I knew then we wouldn't make the 40-60 minute drive to the hospital). But I lied telling Jason that I was fine and could make it! Thank god my eyes were closed 99% of the time and I didn't see the many traffic laws my husband (safely) broke, attempting to get us from Glenview to Oak Park quickly on a Friday morning at 8:45 a.m. in rush hour. We are on I-294, and I get my first expulsive contraction. The type where I'm grunting, uncontrollably pushing. Jason tells me not to push, but I had no choice. (He even pushed my legs together at one point attempting to help me hold him in)! The body does what it wants! I-290 was not an option for travel due to traffic, so Jason went to the local streets. Every 3-5 minutes or so I'm having another bout of pushing without trying. By the time we're in Oak Park—10 minutes from the hospital, 5 minutes from our midwife's office—we decided their office was closer and that's where we were going. Jason called their office several times during this trip. The conversations went from, "We might barely make the hospital" to "NOT AT ALL making the hospital!" I scream "Ring of fire! Ring of fire!" as we are 1 mile from the office. The last 3 blocks I swear I was sitting on Noah's head. Jason turns the corner and pulls up in front of the office (it's technically a "loading zone" but for keeping a good story, we call it a "delivery zone." ☺) He parks the car, opens my door

(I was in the front passenger seat), pulls down my pants and discovers a head emerging. My last contraction begins and he eased our son out of my birth canal and caught him. Noah started crying immediately (thankfully!) and Jason put him on my chest and ran upstairs looking for a midwife to help. Cynthia was already on her way down and they met up on his way back to the car. EMTs were there on standby in case of an emergency, but nothing was needed. They helped us clamp the cord, and accompanied us to the hospital.

Noah Robert Matusiak -born at 9:24 a.m.* in Jason's car. (essentially, a 12-hour labor)

*9/24 is our wedding anniversary and "Wonderful Tonight," our wedding song, was playing on the radio when he was born. NO JOKE.

Now, last but not least, let me share Payton's story with you. He's our third (and last!) baby. After our first 2 hopes of having the "perfect birth" in the relaxing birthing center within the hospital were destroyed, we decided the universe was telling us that having a baby in the hospital was apparently just not for us. So, Payton was a planned home birth. We began working with another midwife practice, Gentle Birth Care in Oak Park, IL, that assisted with home-birth deliveries. May 15, (8 days post "due date") at 7:00 a.m., I woke with the beginnings of labor pain. Eerily similar to the onset of Evan's labor, I was cautiously optimistic as we went about our day to encourage the progression of labor. We even took the boys to the zoo for a few hours hoping that walking around would speed things along. While it did, as soon as I stopped walking, labor would slow down too. So, I knew this was likely going to be longer than Noah's quick 12-hour labor, but hopefully not as long as Evan's! We went back home, and I just wanted to rest. So, I danced the line between walking around to attempt to progress labor, and resting to conserve energy.

Labor moved on all day and night. We had some friends come over to keep our older two occupied while the midwives came to assess my progress around dinnertime. A near repeat of Evan's birth, I was not very far progressed (3-4 cm dilated) after 12 hours of labor. However, there was one main difference this time—I WAS HOME AND HAD NOWHERE TO GO. So I just slept. After learning about the importance of sleep from Noah's experience, I wasn't going to force myself to stay awake throughout labor. My body requires rest to get through it, so that's what I did. Our midwives left around 11:00 p.m. and told us to call them to come back when I knew that things had gotten to a more urgent point. I slept on the couch on and off through contractions, breathing in and out deeply, letting my body give in and surrender to each painful wave. Around 3:30 a.m. I woke up, unable to sleep through contractions any longer. I stumbled over into our room and asked Jason, who was asleep snuggling with Noah (2.5 years old), to call back the midwives. They came back quickly, by 4:00 a.m. I hoped and prayed that when they arrived that I would be close and it would not be a repeat delayed progression like Evan's story. I staggered back to the bed and collapsed as my body was filled with intense pain and emotions. Thankfully, they checked me and I was at 9 cm! My water was still intact, so they offered to break it for me, which would help alleviate the pressure and move things along more quickly. It worked, and shortly after, the contractions intensified more, and I naturally delivered Payton in the comfort of my own bedroom, while leaning against my husband, in a dim-lit relaxing environment. While it was an intense, painful birth, when he was born, he literally cried 2-3 times to open up his lungs, and contentedly nestled onto my chest. It was the most beautiful and serene entrance to the world I had ever experienced.

So, let me explain something here—as dramatic as having a baby in the car was, I'd choose that method of delivery ANY day over the hospital experience I had delivering Evan. Between the lack of sleep, IV fluids, Pitocin, and the epidural, I was very mentally foggy, swollen, and physically drained. After Noah's birth, I felt alert, happy, mentally clear, strong, and empowered. I was ready to embrace visitors and excited to begin the journey of motherhood again. After Payton, while

I felt physically fatigued after 20+ hours of labor and delivery at 4:45 a.m., I felt the deepest sense of love, peace, and calm. Energetically speaking, I can tell you that the differences were not just apparent in *my* symptoms and energy. The differences in my sons' personalities to this day mirror their birth experiences. It may sound like a stretch and that I'm making it up, but to me it's clear. Evan is the most intense and anxious/excitable. Noah is filled with drive and strength. Payton is the most chill and "go with the flow." Now, I understand that these differences could be due to simple personality traits, and/or birth order, but SO MUCH influences our children and their behavior/personality than we can consciously ever know.

When I see patients in my office, at their first visit when we are doing our new patient history and intake appointment, I often ask questions that help me determine their "constitution." I explain that concept this way: we all know someone in our lives that will get sick when someone sneezes from 3 blocks away; at the same time, we know others that if someone would sneeze or vomit ON THEM, they wouldn't bat an eye. We also know those who just "get headaches" as their body's way of communicating when they are overwhelmed and stressed, and others who have digestive upset. We all have an energy—this, "constitution," that influences how and what our bodies will manifest under stressful conditions. This is why I inquire about the patient's history in ways they've likely never experienced before.

"What was your mother's pregnancy like with you?"

"What was your birth experience like?"

"Do you know if you were breastfed, and if so, for how long?"

"Any recurrent infections growing up?"

"Did you have any traumas, emotionally or physically that you recall, or that you were told about, even from an early age?"

These questions essentially lead to conversations about the person's life history, experiences, and personality that affect their mental, emotional, and physical responses to life. How our bodies adapt to external circumstances is a combination of our genetics, parental influence, and energetic implications that began before we were even born. To better understand this concept, I recommend reading Bruce Lipton's book *The Biology of Belief.* There's a chapter toward the end entitled "Conscious Parenting," denoting that parenting truly begins energetically in the time-space continuum before the baby is even born, and to some degree before they were conceived. This may be a stretch for some to grasp. But energy is a real thing, like I mentioned in Chapter 4. This concept extends from who we were (and our experiences and health statuses) before and during our pregnancies, all the way through giving birth and beyond. I don't bring this up to have you worry and overthink every aspect of your pregnancy and delivery story, and get paranoid of how you messed up your baby already. I just had to touch on this topic to create a baseline of awareness of how subtle things that we don't even recognize can create support or imbalance in our lives, our bodies, and our babies, as well!

So, let's finish up this chapter by talking about logistics. I've driven the point home that birth matters—in more ways than we can ever know. Assuming you're like most people, you're reading this already after having had your baby thinking, "Well, too late now! Can't change the past." On the one hand, you're right. On the other hand, simply having that awareness can be helpful as you continue raising your child, <u>and</u> there *might* be a next time. So, that's something to consider if and when you have another baby. (No pressure)!

If you've had a C-section with your first child, frequently doctors will encourage you to just schedule one for your second. Unless they have a legitimate <u>medical</u> reason for recommending this, I believe a VBAC (vaginal birth after cesarean) serves an incredibly important purpose, not only for you and your recovery, but for the baby as well! Did you know that in a vaginal birth, the way the baby emerges through the birth canal is actually responsible for the first inoculation of the bacteria in the baby's gut? It may sound a bit gross, but it's true. As the baby's face is smashed up through the vagina and the rectum of the mother, the normal flora that is present in her nether-regions begins the normal set up of probiotics for baby. The next step of this is breast-feeding as there are bacteria on the mother's skin that are transferred into the child, as well as in the milk. All these bacterium are NORMAL and healthy. Gut imbalances have been shown to be at the root cause of autism spectrum disorders, ADHD, Crohn's, colitis, anxiety, depression, and other inflammatory or immune-based conditions. Proper gut flora is essential to our health as human beings.

So, what happens if we do have a C-section and the baby has missed out on that first opportunity to be introduced to appropriate bacteria for their digestive tract? A few things: 1) Breastfeed if possible. We will discuss this in the next chapter, and any amount of breast-milk, especially from the source, is better than nothing when it comes to baby's gut health! 2) Probiotic supplementation may eventually be necessary as your baby gets older. I don't generally recommend this in young infants, but it can be helpful as baby grows older and depending on other factors. This is a very specific situation that needs to be dealt with one-on-one. 3) If you're by chance reading this before a scheduled C-section, there is something I suggest to mitigate the loss of that inoculation that they would normally receive through a vaginal birth. After the baby has been born, some sources literally recommend wiping through your vagina and rectum with gauze and swabbing the baby's face, mouth, body, and anus with it. This sounds much more disgusting than it needs to be. Just remember, this is exactly what would've happened naturally in a vaginal delivery. I'm not saying to take a chunk of feces and feed it to your child! Please use hygiene and some common sense here. Essentially, whatever you can do in a simple, gentle fashion to simulate coming through the birth canal will be helpful for your growing child.

As I stated when describing Noah's birth story, I was focused on ensuring a lot of chiropractic care during my pregnancy. Regular chiropractic care can be very impactful when it comes to the woman's comfort level and alleviating pains that are common due to ligaments stretching, as they offer less support. However, research also shows that regular care can reduce the duration and discomfort of labor and delivery, also aiding in proper positioning of baby for a smoother transition during birth. As an added benefit to my pregnant patients, at their first postpartum appointment, I encourage them to bring their baby in to receive a complimentary treatment. As described, every birth story is unique and different, potentially presenting a variety of challenges and traumas occurring for both the mother and the child. The sooner and earlier in life that we as holistic healers can intervene and re-establish optimal nervous system function within the body, the less likely your baby will experience the handful of typical issues commonly associated with infants. These are things like: colic, spit up, sleep issues, trouble nursing, and torticollis to name a few.

My son Nathan was an extremely colicky baby, it appeared to be gas related. I started removing items from my diet, but it still continued. I stopped nursing, but it still continued. I tried gripe water, bouncing him softly on a yoga ball, massaging him, but nothing was helping. So I spoke to my husband about seeing Dr. Christy to see if she could help. My husband was reluctant but at this point would try anything and we had our first child visit. In the appointment she took her time to get to know Nathan as a baby and my labor. She then massaged him and did a slight adjustment. We left there unsure if anything worked until Nathan fell asleep for 3 hours, which he never did prior. We panicked and I texted Dr. Christy and she was confident and assured me that something was changing in his body. From the next day forward he was like a completely different child. From that first visit, I bring my kids to see Dr. Christy.
-Kasia D.

Birth can be quite stressful, physically and emotionally. Generally speaking, the more natural state in which we allow it to take place, the less likely there are to be as many shocks to ours and our baby's bodies. Every intervention from IVs, to Pitocin, to epidurals, to C-sections all carry a risk. I highly encourage you to educate yourself a bit on how these procedures became so commonplace, even in seemingly low risk women. The C-section rate in America is approximately 33%. That states that an average of 1 out of every 3 women will have a C-section delivery. Compare this with less than 5% C-section rate in practices with midwives that generally practice with less interference in the birthing process. Remember, cesarean deliveries are SURGERY. Recovery is much longer than with vaginal births, and on top of that, the risks to the baby are much higher as well.

As I said, I'm incredibly grateful that these interventions exist for emergencies. The problem is that, as with many modalities, they are unnecessarily overutilized. If there is ever a next time for you, look into Hypnobabies, Bradley Method, or other natural birthing methods. These institutions excel at preparing your mind and body for a natural birth, and generally speaking, when we are prepared, we are more likely to succeed. Additionally, if a home birth is possible for you, I highly recommend it! There is a lot of misinformation that floats around about its safety. But when you're low risk, it's been proven that home births are safer than hospital births—especially when attended by a qualified professional such as a midwife. My birth with Evan did not go as planned. I'm thankful that I had selected a team of midwives that were there to advocate for me. If I had been with a traditional OB/Gyne practice, I doubt they would've let me labor for 40 hours. I would've ended up with a C-section. The take-home message I learned from all my birth experiences was that we have to empower ourselves with the knowledge and action steps to achieve what we desire. There is no place for fear in the birth process—it's about complete surrender! You and your body are capable of far more than you ever imagined! After all, you created a human—and that was the easy part!

7

Baby's Breastfeeding/ Bottle Feeding Journey

Breast is best.   *and*   *Fed is best.*

Let's talk about boobs! I'm sure you never thought you'd be so excited to read a whole chapter about breasts than since your baby was born, right?! It's pretty common knowledge now that there is no replacement for breastfeeding. The antibodies and immune support, plus the nutritional content that breastmilk provides is unlike anything that we can create in a formula. However, the perspective that "breast is best," also allows us mothers the perfect opportunity to shame ourselves for not being enough. (I know I did for years). This is why I will not judge how one chooses to feed their child. There are so many factors that come into play, and the bottom line is a healthy and happy mom and child. In this chapter we will go through all of the problems and challenges that can occur, and help you through them. My goal is to help you succeed with your breastfeeding journey, no matter what that looks like for you. Because if you don't have the resources or knowledge to handle the hardships, you're more likely to give up.

According to the World Health Organization, only about 40% of infants are still being breastfed by 6 months of age, despite their recommendation to breastfeed exclusively until 6 months, and continue nursing until 24 months. So, if we know its benefits, and the leading authority on health in the world suggests maintaining a breastfeeding relationship for 2 years, why are the majority of women not even making it to 6 months?

I know the reason—breastfeeding is hard! It comes with a variety of challenges. I'll address a handful of them here, and provide some resources to support you. But the biggest problem that I find is the lack of guidance and support. We are taught that breastfeeding is the most natural thing that a mother can do to nourish her child. That's true. However, for most women, it doesn't necessarily come naturally without a substantial amount of work first. I made it despite the odds being stacked way against me. Breastfeeding my kids was nonnegotiable for me. So, I made it work. But as I mentioned earlier, I suffered with severe low supply with all of them. I don't think I ever produced more than 8 ounces in any given day—and that was at BEST, at my maximum, when they had grown a bit and were expected to have about 30 ounces daily. Regardless of that challenge, I nursed all of my boys for over 2 years. I didn't care if they only got 1 ounce a day from me, they were going to get it. Now at the same time, my sanity may have suffered as a result of that determination. And of course, that is the decision we all have to weigh with regard to our priorities and what we believe we have the emotional capacity to handle. But let's go through all the information about why I feel breastfeeding is worth the hassle.

It's amazing how nature provided such a perfect food for our little ones. Breastmilk (AKA liquid gold) delivers your baby an abundant amount of enzymes, antioxidants, antibodies, nutrients, and calming compounds in an easily absorbable way. The most amazing part is that it's constantly changing daily to give your baby exactly what he/she needs at that specific point in their development. Our bodies are exposed to viruses/bacteria all day, and we mount an immune response to all those challenges and pass that immune support to our babies through our milk, protecting them from infections. Additionally, your milk composition will look substantially different between nursing your 6-week-old, vs. your 6-month-old. This is exactly why women can tandem breastfeed a toddler and their newborn, and each child somehow gets milk designed specifically for them. That is pretty incredible to me! Breastfed babies generally have stronger immune systems, therefore, they experience fewer colds, ear infections, or cases of meningitis; lower incidence of SIDS (sudden infant death syndrome); fewer digestive imbalances (colic, reflux, diarrhea, or constipation); fewer childhood cancers; fewer skin issues/allergies; lowered obesity rates as they grow; and even better vision. I encourage you to do a Google search for a picture from a biology student in England that illustrates petri dishes completely colonized with bacteria, except in the center where a drop of breastmilk clearly inhibited the growth. It's fascinating! I wish I could include it here, but couldn't for copyright reasons...so check it out! ☺

Besides all the benefits nursing provides your baby, the positives exist for us moms, too! Mothers who have breastfed generally have a lowered incidence of breast and ovarian cancers, autoimmune conditions, endometriosis, heart disease, osteoporosis, and diabetes. Emotionally, studies show that due to the hormonal influx required to breastfeed, nursing mothers are apparently calmer, happier, have higher confidence, and less anxiety/postpartum depression. And here's the thing that, in my opinion, is the most important of all—it allows for a deep connection with your baby that is so exceptional and unique, that nothing else in the world can compare. Looking into your baby's eyes, snuggling them against your chest skin-to-skin as they drink your milk is literally the most beautiful thing on the planet. Of course this is not to say that one cannot adequately bond with a baby through bottle-feeding—dads, grandparents and other friends/relatives do this all the time. It's just not the same. That connection transcends time, space, and anything tangible from the physical world.

As beautiful as it is when it works well, it sucks (no pun intended) when it doesn't. Here are some of the most common issues that women are faced with when working on breastfeeding.

LIP/TONGUE TIES

Have you ever heard a lactation consultant tell you that breastfeeding shouldn't hurt? They're right, sort of. When you're first starting out, it is absolutely normal for it to take some time for your body to adjust to a small human gnawing on your nipples for hours a day. The early days of nursing are you acclimating to your baby, learning to latch them properly, and holding them in the most comfortable way for you. I met with plenty of lactation consultants in my early days, and latch usually wasn't my problem. But, it still hurt getting used to constant suckling. When Evan was 4 days old, he pulled off my breast abruptly and took with it a chunk of skin, causing my nipple to bleed! That wasn't pleasant! Nursing hurt for some time, even though his latch was fine. But they are right, that after you get used to it, there should never be a sharpness of pain.

So, after the first few weeks of navigating the nursing relationship with your little one, those kinks should be getting worked out a bit. You'll become aware of the difference between pain from over stimulation that you're just dealing with, versus pain from a bad latch or something being wrong. The metaphor I use is that of post-workout soreness. It is normal and expected after starting a new exercise routine or getting back into one after some time off. This type of pain ("good" pain) is VERY different than the sharpness of an injury that causes you to stop in your tracks or move with a limp or other compensations. Trust yourself and your body to communicate with you that something isn't right if you're experiencing "bad" pain nursing.

Tongue and lip ties are incredibly common now. They are diagnosed when an abnormally short frenulum (the piece of skin that connects the tongue to the mouth underneath or the lip to the gum line) restricts the tongue's ability to function properly. When they are severe enough, they can limit a proper latch and cause pain and blisters or "blebs" to form on your nipples. An improper latch due to a tie not only can cause pain and discomfort for the mother, but also poor milk transfer that can result in slow weight gain and low milk supply. Many lactation consultants are trained to look for this, but it is best corrected with laser therapy by a pediatric dentist. As opposed to scalpel from an ENT doctor, pediatric dentists are experts in this issue, and can get you a proper diagnosis, as they are easily missed otherwise. I'll include resources for this at the end.

I kept thinking, "maybe it just takes awhile for them to get the hang of it." I struggled for weeks and weeks with excruciating pain every time he latched. Add insult to injury, he wasn't gaining weight and my doctors were threatening to put him in the hospital. What more could I do?! I was already nursing around the clock, supplementing formula as necessary. And the doctors had no answers. The first person to discover that my son had a lip and tongue tie, was actually his pediatric chiropractor. Once it was revised, and he latched for the first time after the procedure, I literally cried tears of joy. I wasn't crazy. I felt an immediate difference, and suddenly he was gaining and I no longer had to supplement his feeds. In my research, I learned ties can also impact speech, and other components of health, such as tension in the neck/jaw, headaches, and behavior as they grow older. Doctors at the hospital told me to just feed him from a bottle, which to me was avoiding the underlying issue. Luckily when my second son was born, I had already educated myself enough and was more experienced in nursing my oldest for 22 months, so I was more able to nurse effectively and navigate around the lip tie even before getting it revised. Anyway, I just want to tell women that while it's challenging, it's absolutely

*possible to nurse even when your child has a tie. But get it revised
by a pediatric dentist ASAP!*
-Amanda M.

LOW SUPPLY

Low supply is WAY more common than Dr. Google would have
you believe. It's why I waited so long to supplement Evan's feeds, because I thought I "couldn't possibly" be one of the 5% or fewer that
had "true" low supply. For some, there are natural ways of improving
your supply. For others, like myself, there may be nothing you can do.
Some women may appear to have low supply because the baby has a lip
or tongue tie as discussed above, and once the latch is corrected, milk
flows better and your baby can gain weight more easily. If that is the
case, then weighing your baby before and after feeding will be able to
tell you as such. If you can pump 3–4 ounces at a time, but comparing
pre-/post- feeding, your baby only gained/transferred 1.5 ounces, there
is likely something wrong with his or her latch or ability to transfer the
milk properly. This is where IBCLCs (Internationally Board Certified
Lactation Consultants) excel and support you.

I believe I suffered from a condition called "IGT"—Insufficient
Glandular Tissue. This means that for whatever reason, hormonal or
genetic, during puberty, my breast tissue didn't develop properly, and
there just weren't enough ducts created, or tissue available to create
milk in the appropriate amount. Women that suffer from this generally have little to no breast changes during pregnancy. While most
pregnant women see their size double or triple during pregnancy, and
even more once their milk comes in, my breasts didn't really change
at all. Aside from quantity being manufactured as an issue, the rate
in which the breast refills is commonly an issue with IGT. I learned
through a lot of my research when I was searching for my own answers
on why my breasts failed me, a lot of breastfeeding success has to do

with metabolic health of the mother. Polycystic Ovarian Syndrome, Diabetes, Hypothyroidism, and more can influence your milk supply. Being on the birth control pill for almost 7 years really impacted my hormones negatively, and I am sure it had a lot to do with my issues as well.

I consumed all the teas, all the fenugreek, drank gallons of water—and I'll share all those secrets with you here. But if you have IGT, rarely anything helps. But guess what??? Even though I didn't produce more than 5-8 ounces per day, I never gave up. I supplemented, but pumped for over a year with all 3 and nursed them all for over 2 years. If *I* can continue and persevere, so can you!!! The good news is that my situation is rare. It's not impossible, but not highly likely. If you feel like you may have this situation, I recommend reaching out to an International Board Certified Lactation Consultant (IBCLC), and checking out the Facebook group that saved my sanity and connected me with other women who not only struggled like I did to produce milk, but also CARED enough to work to improve it. I would also suggest potentially looking into a supplemental nursing system (SNS), if your supply is so low that it's nearly impossible to breastfeed even a little bit. If you still want the experience of nursing and closeness in that way without the ability to produce, an SNS allows you to supplement with whatever is needed, but through a small tube taped to your chest. I never used one but I know several mothers who have done so with great success.

Let's say for sake of argument that you're not one that has severe milk supply like me. The odds are in your favor—the majority of women CAN breastfeed; it just takes work and listening to your body. Making enough milk is a game of supply and demand. The more the baby nurses and demands milk, the more your body will make. Aside from on-demand feeding, being certain to drink enough water is critical! I frequently suggest a gallon of water per day for breastfeeding moms. Eating enough is also important because if you're malnourished, your body won't be capable of milk production in adequate quantity either.

So, assuming you're in the "average" camp of breastfeeding mothers, we know that regulating breastmilk supply is a simple supply and demand game. This is why if you try to put your baby on a feeding schedule too soon, your supply will likely tank. I always recommend nursing your baby "on demand" for the first few months. This means literally anytime your baby makes a peep, put your breast in his/her mouth. This not only is teaching your body to make milk constantly, but it simultaneously provides the comfort and safety your baby needs to develop trust and connection with you in those early days. Win-Win! The trick is to be sure that first and foremost your baby has a healthy productive latch. This is why I recommend every baby within the first week of birth be evaluated by an IBCLC. They will evaluate them for lip and tongue ties, check latch, position, and provide you the tips needed to ensure that baby is getting what they need from you.

Also, I suggest investing in a few rental items if you feel you're not producing what your baby needs. 1) Hospital grade breast pump. They are worth it—gentle, yet stronger and better than any pump you can get from the store. This way you can get an idea for how much you actually produce. However, that can also be deceiving because, although rare, some women don't respond well to the pump. 2) Baby scale. This way you can do pre-and post- feeding weighs to assess what the baby transfers from you. I'm sure you've read and heard from many other sources that the primary signs to look for to determine if baby is getting enough food is to count wet diapers and to check their weight gain. This is absolutely correct, so I won't reinvent the wheel with how to tell if your baby is hydrated. Another way to notice, however, is to look for the presence of uric acid crystals in your baby's diaper. This is also known as "brick dust." It is a reddish/orangeish colored tint in the urine. This can indicate dehydration. It is not of urgent cause for concern, but one must assess it combined with other factors, like baby's disposition, number of wet diapers, baby's age, etc. The general rule of thumb in the beginning is wet diapers should be equal to the number of days old the child is: day 1 = 1 wet diaper, day 2 = 2 wet diapers, days 3-5= 3-5 wet diapers. By a week old they should have at least 6–8 wet diapers daily.

Essentially, unless you have IGT, or another substantial reason for not producing enough milk, expect it to take about 2 months to find a groove to your feeding routine and schedule. Once again, I advise feeding on demand for the first 6-12 weeks to fully establish a full supply and reproducible system. "Scheduling feeds" too early can be detrimental to their growth, your supply, and the relationship that is being built in those early months. It won't be easy, especially not in the beginning when you're still learning the process and how your baby will adapt. But don't give up! It ends up much easier in the long run. If you're experiencing some low supply I encourage the following:

- ✓ Drink close to a gallon of water daily!
- ✓ Keep your calorie intake high! (Don't forget to feed yourself in the midst of feeding your small human!)
- ✓ Drink "mother's milk tea!"
- ✓ Keep your blood sugar balanced by choosing healthy, nutrient dense foods!
- ✓ Get adequate rest! (as much as possible!)

Enjoy lactation supportive foods (galactogogues) within moderation as alcohol and grains tend to stress blood sugar, which can have the opposite effect on milk supply. Some of these galactogogues include: Guinness beer, oats, barley, fennel, fenugreek, brewer's yeast, chickpeas, almonds, dark leafy greens (kale, spinach, broccoli, alfalfa), ginger, garlic, and papaya.

OVERSUPPLY

I used to be jealous of women who produced too much milk, as I never produced enough. But I understand that the struggle is real for so many. While it wasn't my issue, I know it can be just as difficult to maintain a successful breastfeeding relationship when your breasts are overfilled, leaking, and painful. I've known many women whose babies could not keep up with their flow, and would choke and gag due to their oversupply. After the first month or so, your baby will likely learn to manage the flow and amount of milk. But it can be very challenging in the beginning to navigate this.

Here are a few signs that you may have an oversupply:

- Your baby can't keep up with your let down and cries at your breast as your milk is flowing.
- You experience painful engorgement that isn't relieved by your baby nursing on both sides.
- Your baby has excessive spit up.

When managing oversupply, you clearly should avoid doing anything in the previous section that will support extra milk. Additionally, some techniques to utilize are laid-back nursing to reduce the flow force, and block nursing. Block nursing is when you pick a time frame with which to only nurse from one breast. (for example 3–4 hours). Then switch sides for the same interval. Within a few days, your body should begin to adjust to the lessened demand from both sides and reduce the amount of milk being produced. Remember, when you get uncomfortable, you can hand express or pump just to the point of comfort, and then stop. The more you drain the breast, the more your body gets the message to make more.

Before you try ice packs, the google-recommended cabbage leaves, and the above methods to slow production down, you want to be really sure that baby has a pattern of regularly gaining weight, producing wet and dirty diapers, and that you still have leftover milk. For some women, this may be a good thing. If you need to prepare for going back to work, you may want to pump after feedings to develop a good freezer stash for your caregiver to feed your child when you need to leave him/her. However, I RARELY recommend this practice until after your child is at least 2–3 weeks old. Remember, increasing demand will increase your supply. If you won't need a freezer stash, after a few weeks of getting through it, you can do what I call "pumping to comfort." Basically, after a feeding if you're still feeling full, you may pump just to the point of feeling better, and then stopping. You have to find the balance that works for you—and I'm not going to pretend I am a lactation consultant. This is absolutely their domain, and as I said before, I believe all babies/mothers should meet with an IBCLC within the 1st week of life to identify potential struggles, and offer guidance and solutions as early as possible.

I will say this for anyone out there that would be interested—due to my significant low supply, my babies were lucky enough to grow with the assistance of milk donations from women in the oversupply crowd. If you have the time, desire, and patience to do so, breastmilk donation is, in my opinion, one of the most amazing gifts one can provide a struggling mother. I can't thank my donors enough for the gift they gave my kids—pure, quality, breastmilk so I didn't have to turn to formula for supplementation. Donation sites on Facebook are easy to find—Human Milk for Human Babies, and Eats on Feets were the two local connections I used when I didn't know anyone personally.

CLOGGED DUCTS

This is definitely a common problem in those with oversupply, but I was a victim of clogged ducts frequently as well. They are painfully agonizing— just what you want to experience after enduring childbirth! There are several reasons one might be susceptible to a clogged duct:

Incorrect latch – If the baby isn't transferring milk well, and therefore leaves milk behind in the breast, it can easily block the ducts.

Engorgement and oversupply – This is why I don't recommend "scheduling" feedings early on. You want the baby to empty the breasts frequently to establish a good supply and routine, but also to keep the flow of milk frequent enough to prevent clogs.

Restrictive bras or clothing – Pressure on the breast from a tight bra or wire can impact the flow of milk and cause a clog.

Dehydration – Obviously you want to stay well hydrated for good supply and flow of milk.

Salt deficiency – Maintaining an adequate level of sodium in your diet is important to avoid "stickiness" throughout to prevent plugged ducts.

My solutions to these problems are simple. Prevention above all else is important!

1. I'll say it <u>again</u> – get the opinion of an IBCLC to evaluate latch to be sure the cause of the clogged duct is not baby's latch and lack of milk transfer.
2. Be sure to feed regularly on demand to reduce the likelihood of engorgement and buildup of milk.
3. Avoid snug bras and clothing for long periods of time. I literally LIVED in my nursing tank for at least a year for comfort and ease.
4. Be sure you're drinking AT LEAST half your body weight in ounces of water daily—if you can get closer to a gallon each day, even better!

5. Take an organic sunflower lecithin supplement daily—I recommend 3,000-5,000 mg/day for prevention, and more spread out throughout the day to treat a current clog.

6. Do the salt test to determine if you need more salt daily.

The Salt Test
This was a suggestion from my first pediatrician, Dr. Peter Rosi. Salt can help keep the milk from being too sticky and thick, similar to the supplement I recommend (Sunflower Lecithin). And if you are salt deficient, it can easily lead to clogs, just as frequently as if you were dehydrated. So, daily, do this test. Take a bite of your food without salt. Then, follow it up with another bite of food with a healthy amount of standard table salt on it. Salt naturally by itself tastes bad, so if the salted bite tastes better to you, you're likely salt deficient and need to supplement/add salt liberally to your food. I suggest pink Himalayan salt as it has the highest mineral content and is therefore the healthiest kind you can find. If the unsalted bite tastes worse, then your salt status is likely ok.

You'd be surprised how common it is to be salt deficient. The reason is that our adrenal glands (little glands that sit on top of our kidneys) are responsible for all the stress in our lives no matter where it comes from. Emotionally, physically, nutritionally, etc. When we become depleted, and our adrenals slow their output of various hormones, things become imbalanced. One of those hormones is cortisol, which many of us know has implications for inflammation, stress, weight gain, and more. A less commonly known hormone is aldosterone— this is responsible for a series of reactions that essentially ends with having the kidneys reabsorb sodium and water. Not enough aldosterone will lead to you peeing out all your water, resulting in dehydration and a salt deficiency. Correcting your adrenal imbalance and therefore managing your stress is critical to addressing this issue long term. But in the short term, while we know that as a new mother stress will be a staple for you, you can be conscious of adequate salt and water intake. I recommend checking in on your "salt status" daily.

It is important to treat a clogged duct fast so that it doesn't advance and turn into mastitis, a breast infection that can make you deeply sick. Warm compresses and massage were my "go-to" every time I had a clog. Sometimes recommendations have been to use a fine-toothed comb in the shower to push and try to break up the clog. Additionally, shaking the breast laterally and up/down can be helpful. Pushing tons of water, as well as "dangle nursing" can enlist gravity's assistance in pulling the clog out. This is where your baby lays down and you simply dangle your breast over them to nurse. If not utilizing that position, pointing their nose towards the painful blockage helps them target the affected area better, as well. So nurse/pump as frequently as possible on the affected side to assist in removing the block. With a lot of dedicated (and painful!) work, it will loosen up and improve within a few days. The other things I have found that help a lot is salt intake, (as discussed above with the salt test) and sunflower lecithin. You can take lecithin for prevention of clogged ducts (3,000 mg daily, or more if recurrent). In treatment of an acute clog, I've had patients take over 10,000 mg in a day before. Lecithin is a phospholipid that has both fatty and watery components to it. Therefore, it is thought to prevent and treat plugged milk ducts by increasing the fatty acids in the milk that reduces its stickiness and thickness. If you take too much, you may experience some stomach discomfort or diarrhea. Otherwise, overdosing is harmless. But just monitor the condition closely as mastitis can be serious.

MASTITIS

An untreated clogged duct can easily turn into mastitis. This is when the breast becomes acutely painful, red, swollen, and warm.

Frequently, it can involve an infection. When this occurs, you may have a fever associated with your symptoms as well. During these cases, an antibiotic is usually warranted. However, I have successfully treated mastitis in myself and patients before without antibiotics. Homeopathy, as we will discuss again in later chapters, can be VERY impactful when you get the right remedy. Belladonna 30C is classic for an acute red hot mastitis that is accompanied with a fever. When treating it this way, I suggest taking 4 pellets of Belladonna 30C under your tongue and letting them dissolve completely. You actually hold the tube upside down, twist the cap, and when the pellets fall out, you remove the cap and dump the pellets directly underneath your tongue so you don't have to touch them with your fingers. Our skin has oils that can diminish the potency of homeopathy. Repeat this every 15 minutes for an hour. If after a few hours of this procedure, there is no change, then I would of course not mess around and call your doctor for an appointment and likely an antibiotic prescription. However, it is worth trying for a short time to correct it without drugs. No medication is without risk, but homeopathy is the safest we can find. Antibiotics will pass through to the baby and mess with your gut and the baby's. So if you can avoid them, that is great!

MILK BLISTERS ("BLEBS")

A lip or tongue tie or improper latch can lead to the development of "blebs" on or around your nipple. Essentially, these are painful and blister-like, and frequently look like a tiny white or yellow spot about the size of a pin head on your nipple. It looks similar to a small pimple with a white head. The white or yellow color is from milk that is trapped inside the overgrown skin on top of a duct/opening. Sometimes they aren't painful, and if not, that makes correcting them all the easier. Treatment of milk blisters and blebs is nearly identical to that of clogged ducts. I often encourage massage and rubbing coconut oil into the area as well. Providing the affected tissue with massage, lubrication, and warmth helps to loosen the hardened milk inside, and liberates it to get things flowing again. Topical coconut oil (and breast-milk for that matter!) is highly functional as it also helps to prevent/treat infections as both have antiviral, and antibacterial properties.

THRUSH

Thrush is a fungal infection that can develop on your breast and get transferred back and forth between your breast and your baby. That makes it somewhat challenging to treat effectively and quickly in some advanced cases. Antifungal topical creams are the standard of care. However, my first recommendation is to use coconut oil topically on your breasts frequently, especially before/after feeds. It is safe to con-tinue breastfeeding through thrush, but depending on the severity of the infection, it can be rather painful. Another remedy besides coconut oil is a simple vinegar wash. As long as your breasts and nipples are not cracked, you can dilute a tablespoon of apple cider vinegar (ACV) in a cup of water, and use that solution to rinse and cleanse the area. The benefit of ACV and coconut oil topically is that you don't have to worry about latching and nursing your baby after applying it as they are completely safe. With other antifungal medications, it's usually en-couraged to wipe the area clean before breastfeeding as many are not intended for internal use and can be harmful if swallowed.

My most important take-home message when I've treated women and their babies with thrush is the importance of diet and proper gut flora balance. Thrush is caused by yeast fungus—Candida albicans. Candida lives normally on our skin and in our digestive tract, and only becomes a problem when there is an overgrowth causing an infection. Sugar feeds Candida and will cause the death of the "good" bacteria that keep the yeast and "bad" bacteria in check. Therefore, eliminating sugar from the diet is critical in treatment and prevention. Probiotic supplementation in the mom, and sometimes the baby, depending on the situation will also be helpful. If your thrush seems severe and not healing within a week or two, I highly suggest contacting your trusted practitioner.

BOTTLE FEEDING AND "NIPPLE CONFUSION"

For moms that go back to work, and have to continue pumping and providing bottles while away, many fear that the baby will get "nipple confused" and refuse the breast when getting used to the nipple on a bottle. The truth is that "nipple confusion" doesn't actually exist. A nipple is a nipple to a baby. What happens sometimes when a baby starts to refuse your breast after bottle feeding is what I refer to as "flow preference." Generally speaking, bottle feeds allow the milk to flow more quickly than it would naturally from your breast. So, when babies become accustomed to this speed of eating, they grow less patient and more frustrated when nursing. This in turn, frustrates and tires us moms out, and then we begin weaning from nursing sooner than intended.

There is an easy solution to prevent this from occurring if you're committed to continuing your nursing relationship, while also utilizing bottle feeding. Even if you are not breastfeeding and only bottle feeding, it's a useful technique I promote to encourage your baby to take his/her time with their feeds. It's called "paced feeding." To perform a paced feed, you sit your baby up more so than laying them cradled. This way you can keep the bottle parallel to the floor, and slowly give a little bit of milk at a time. Encourage them to suck a bit first, as they would at the breast to elicit a let-down. Many have a concern that the baby will suck too much air and get a stomachache. This is not typically the case as you don't let them swallow air for more than a few seconds before allowing milk to flow. Burping also usually takes care of this; so, while it's something to be conscious of, I wouldn't worry about it.

Using the slowest flow of a nipple regardless of the baby's age will also support the continuation of the nursing relationship. This bottle feeding technique is slower, averaging in the baby taking about an ounce every 5–10 minutes, depending on their age. As they get older, it will speed up. This system takes a lot of patience, but I truly believe it is worth it, if it's important to you to continue breastfeeding when you're present, but you need to give bottles whether to supplement feeds, or for caregivers to provide your baby while you're away.

Paced bottle feeding is something really easy to YouTube a tutorial. This system allows the baby to control their pace, and avoids them overfeeding, too. You can also encourage him/her to pause throughout the feeding by gently removing the nipple out of their mouth, and angling the bottle down so they won't get milk. When they are still hungry, they will make it clearly known that they weren't done and keep sucking, to which you then carefully level it back up to allow milk to flow again. The most important part is to hold the bottle closer to horizontally and parallel to the floor, as compared to traditional bottle feeding. You can compare the following pictures.

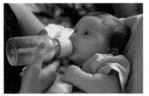 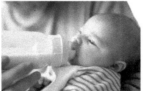 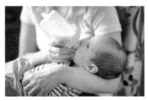

Paced feed style   *Paced feed style*   *Inclined, not paced*

I know the majority of what I discussed here was nursing related. This is just such an important topic, and I assume that based on the stats, most women want to breastfeed, but stop due to struggles and not enough resources and support to continue on. I want to be that support for you. If you need to or decide to do formula, you should know that they are not all created equal. I always recommend finding an organic variety and/or a goat's milk-based kind. Cow's milk often elicits allergic responses. In an effort to provide hypoallergenic formulas, many companies then offer a soy type as well. This is even worse in my opinion as it wreaks havoc on the child's hormones. I encourage you to look up Holle and Hipp formulas. They are the highest quality brands of formula that I know, although they aren't available commercially in the U.S. I've also included a link in the resources from the Weston Price Foundation that has a recipe for making homemade formula, as well!

Here are some final thoughts regarding nursing/bottle feeding/pumping/formula feeding your baby—Breast may be "best," but ultimately what is best, is a fed, happy baby, and a balanced healthy mom. I fought tooth and nail to breastfeed my kids despite not making enough milk, and I'm very glad I did. But it did not come without challenges, heartache, and exhaustion. Whatever you choose, I encourage you to own your decision with peace. Forget what others say or think. Your choices are your choices. I am a passionate breastfeeding advocate, but NOT at the expense of your mental health. Trying to nurse with obstacles can easily turn into an obsession of counting ounces, and weighing feeds that takes away from connecting with your sweet little cherub. We are human. Give yourself grace in this journey and take one day at a time. Any time spent breastfeeding and any ounces given to your baby are a gift, and as we addressed in the first chapter, your sanity is also a gift. ☺ I've given you a lot of resources to persevere through challenges, if that's your choice. I encourage you to evaluate your priorities, what you want, and why you want it. Then you can make a clear decision to support yourself and your baby's health.

8

Baby's Food Foundation

"The food you eat can either be the most powerful form of
medicine, or the slowest form of poison."
-Ann Wigmore

It's time to talk about building your child's health through the foundation of his/her diet. If you were able to persevere through breastfeeding, you've already set a stage for them in the healthiest way imaginable. Remember, everything you were able to give was a gift. Whether that was 2 days, 2 years, or longer. Now, I never recommend starting your baby on solid foods before 6 months of age. This is for a few reasons. 1) Their guts are not ready to begin digesting any foods except breastmilk/formula until at least this time – usually longer. (you'll notice food come out as it goes in due to this exact reason)! 2) Developmentally, your baby is not ready for eating solid foods until at least 6 months. Your baby must be capable of sitting up on his/her own before it is safe to begin. If you let your baby be your guide, they will instruct you on what is best on their timetable.

I strongly believe in setting the proper foundation for kids early on. Even though their body isn't reliant on nutrients from their foods at this point, you have an opportunity to set the stage of their palate for what foods they come to enjoy and crave. We as adults come to assume that babies and children are picky eaters and don't like healthy foods.

This couldn't be farther from the truth! Kids eat what they know. If all we feed them in their early years are sugars, starches, and refined foods, that's all they will come to expect, and become picky eaters. Then our expectations become a reality and the idea that "kids don't like vegetables" exists because of how they were taught. My kids always ate very well from early on. And I'll explain the system we utilized to encourage them to become independent and healthy eaters. But first and foremost we must stop prejudging what babies will/will not like based on our own biases and taste buds! In all honesty, the healthier <u>we</u> eat, the healthier our babies will eat. This is an excellent opportunity for you to eat healthfully yourself. We are the leaders—so, if all we eat is pizza, chocolate, and fries, that is what our small humans will desire as well. We lead by example.

But, can I tell you a secret? We actually set the stage even before our babies are born, based on how we ate during our pregnancy with them. Our diet changes the flavor of the amniotic fluid and they can energetically and nutritionally pick up on all that we did while they were still inside us developing. They get used to food quality in the womb and those patterns can absolutely translate into their preferences as they grow. What we eat during our pregnancies has a REAL impact on their growth, development, health, and vitality. In fact, I can share a story with you that actually happened and scared me to my very core...

I was on vacation when I was about 7 months pregnant with Evan. I was visiting some family in Arizona, and while I was far from perfect with regard to eating healthy, I was very health conscious when compared to my family. But, I was on vacation and so I wasn't concerned for a few days. I let go, as many of us do when we are away, and had more than my fair share of sugar/snacks/junk—in the form of donuts, ice cream, bagels, refined carbohydrates, etc. Well, after about 3 days of that, I realized for a day *that I hadn't felt him move. I thought maybe I was hallucinating, and just being paranoid. I truly didn't have a sense that anything was <u>really</u> wrong, but it was certainly unnerving that at 7 months pregnant I hadn't felt the familiar (albeit sometimes annoying, and painful) kicks, punches and feet poking my spleen. The entire day, I was acutely aware and micromanaging any sensation that could've been construed as baby movements. If there were some happening, they were so light and subtle that I barely noticed. That evening we went out to dinner at an Italian restaurant, and while everyone else enjoyed pizza and pasta dishes, I trusted my gut and ordered salmon and broccoli. My body was beginning to feel really crappy from all the indulgences and I needed a break! Within an hour, I was greeted again with bouncing kicks and movement inside me. No. Joke. My message? He was PISSED that I fed him nothing but crap for the week and was essentially drugged and tired. Lesson learned the hard way. My point is that this foundation is truly set long before actually introducing solids.*

I'll share my solid introducing method in a moment, but I wanted to share one other thing first. Concurrently with this process, I found the greatest teether EVER! A cool, crisp, raw, organic cucumber! It was amazing! Especially when they are still just teething and cannot bite off a chunk yet, my kids just gnawed the heck out of the cucumber to the point where they would get some of the natural flavor and juices out of it. Same thing with a full-size, raw, organic carrot. The real natural food feels good on their gums, and nutritionally they are getting some benefit from it too!

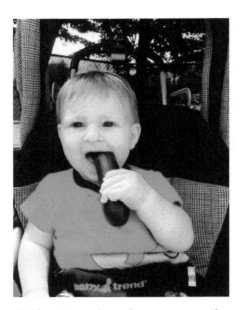

Noah at 8 months teething on a cucumber

So, let's talk about introducing first foods. Many people assume the only way is to either buy premade purees, or to make your own. Making your own can be very time consuming. But buying them calls into question the quality of what you're purchasing. Is there a better way? In my opinion, yes! It's called baby-led weaning (BLW). If you haven't heard about this method of food introduction, let me explain. This process actually starts long before your baby is ready to begin solids. *Observation* is the first step. They are watching what, how, and when you eat. They watch your patterns, and learn social cues from meal times. They learn manners (kinda), haha! I know I can't be the only one that sat and nursed my child at the dinner table eating over his head. Mama has to eat too, and you KNOW that as soon as you want to sit and eat, your baby has radar and wakes from their nap and demands to eat or be held! Who can blame them?! Meals are a social time in our culture, and they just want to be a part of the family dynamic. So, they've been observing for 6 months. Then, when they hit

6 months, you can keep them in your lap (or if they are ready, in a high chair) and you give them their first option for their own food that doesn't come from a breast or a bottle. But it's not their own blend of purees that is different from what everyone is eating. It's what you're eating. You obviously have to be cautious about textures to ensure their safety. But it's usually pretty simple to cut up some of the cooked vegetables off your plate to start. (Hence, this is why you eating healthy is the first step to growing a healthy child!)

This method of introducing food teaches them to rely on themselves for feeding, which is great for them, but also for you! You don't have to waste half of your own meal time feeding him/her. You can enjoy your meal! This is the chance for your baby to learn and explore textures, tastes, chewing, their tongue, hand-mouth coordination, and swallowing something other than liquid. There is a quote that says, "food before 1 is just for fun." It's mainly correct, as they are getting all they need nutritionally from breastmilk or formula. Introducing foods is a stage in their development. Learning to eat is a skill they will use the rest of their life. It is great to start between 6 to 9 months of age as this is where their interest typically peaks. In some families with a strong nursing relationship, a baby will play and enjoy trying foods for awhile, and after establishing pincer grasp and understanding how it works, they go back to exclusively nursing again. This didn't happen for any of my kids, as my boys love to eat!!

There are two components to this process of BLW. *How* your child is learning to eat, and *what* they are eating. So, let's continue with the how—after the purely observation stage has been completed, you allow baby to feed themselves by presenting him/her with a few bites of softened table food. It is unnecessary for you to put it in their mouth for them. When they are ready, they will do this themselves. Remember, this is also teaching independence, which you'll be grateful for in the coming months. In my experience, 6-7 month olds are just intrigued with the process and grab at the food, but may not eat it. Some may end up on the floor, some in their hair. Rarely will it end up in their mouth. But this is a part of their self-discovery process. If you get impatient (as I did, too—don't worry this does not have to be an all or nothing kind of thing), you may put a piece of the food in their mouth to show them how it's done. Most of the time, they will look confused and not know what to do with it. But over time, usually between 7 to 8 months of age, they start to get the hang of things on their own. They develop the pincer grasp so they gain better control and dexterity over what they pick up and can get into their mouths. It is actually an amazing experience to watch a child go through their own stages of this process and figure it out. By 9 months, many babies who have started with BLW are completely eating independently at a table with the family. It takes the pressure off you of having to force feed them strained peas. No airplane noises. They have come to learn that meal time is a social experience and you teach appropriate food behavior at this time as well.

My method was to always begin with cooked vegetables. This was easy for us, as we always had a vegetable with every meal. Soft, grasp-able cubes of food that you can put out for them to "feed themselves" is the best way to go. Here is a list of my kids' "first" foods: avocado, cooked carrots, zucchini, sweet potato, butternut squash, and cauliflower. These foods are soft, simple textures that can be cut up into small bites. You place a few cubes out at a time, and let your baby have free reign. Some will jump in immediately. Others won't seem interested. Either is ok! Just like anything else, food is best introduced when they are truly ready. Some babies will be interested but take awhile to actually learn how to get food from their hand into their mouth. This is a process—and it's one that your baby has to learn on his/her own. Giving some assistance and showing them that food is good to go in their mouth is fine. I just mean that spoon-feeding a baby can create laziness and a sense of passiveness with regard to meals. If they take an active role in the process, their reward centers in the brain will light up and provide them with continued incentive to keep working on it.

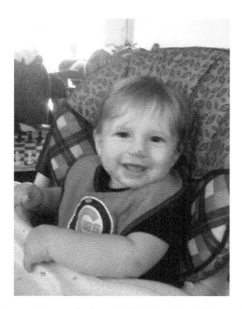

Evan at 9 months happily feeding himself avocado

The next foods I focused on introducing were more complex textures, yet still more vegetables, such as: cooked broccoli, asparagus, green beans, etc. Notice that I haven't mentioned some incredibly common first foods like bananas and rice cereal. Here's why. Rice cereal is nutritionally void. It is essentially a useless food, and the advice of older generations recommending to put it in your baby's bottle to help him/her sleep longer is outdated, and quite frankly dangerous. Not to mention the fact that the levels of arsenic in rice are measurably higher than most adults should be consuming regularly, let alone your infant! Bananas on the other hand may surprise you. They are soft. A perfect texture. A whole food, high in vitamins and minerals. Why wouldn't I start my kids with bananas?! I didn't introduce ANY fruits in my babies until they were over 9-10 months old. As I mentioned at the beginning of this chapter, introducing foods is about setting the foundation of their palate and taste buds. Bananas and most fruits are very high in sugar. Natural sugar, but still sugar. Begin with things that they may refuse if they don't get used to it first. Let's be honest, it'll be rare that you feed a banana or other sweet food that they don't like. First foods are paramount. You truly have a golden opportunity to have your kid enjoy healthy food. Don't rob them of that chance. They are going to likely want and enjoy sugar the rest of their lives. If they start with bananas and applesauce, I can nearly guarantee they will never be interested in zucchini. What's the point of that flavor when they could have something tastier?! This is why my suggestion is to wait on introducing fruits. Set a strong foundation so they will enjoy vegetables first, and then expand their palate to include other foods.

I began giving proteins like softer meats, fish, and eggs even before fruits. Baby gums are just as sharp if not sharper than many adult teeth. If you've ever nursed a teething baby when they clamp down, you know this to be true! Even if they don't yet have teeth, they can still learn to chew! Another concern many parents have utilizing this method is the worry about the baby choking. There are a few pieces of good news here. The gag reflex is located much farther forward in their mouth than older children and adults. This is purposeful by nature. As the baby learns to navigate solid foods, they will gag and learn how to move their tongue and mouth to eat the food properly. Gagging does not mean they are choking. The gag reflex is *protective* against choking. I did this process with all 3 of my boys, and not once did any of them choke on their food. There were a few instances of gagging, and watchful observation to be sure they figured out how to maneuver the food well, and each time they learned on their own.

So, you may be asking now, did I EVER use purees with my babies? Yes. I did. But it was the exception and not the rule. Sometimes I pureed things myself, but more often I just bought organic purees from the store. But, quite honestly, it was easier to simply give them what we had cooked for our own meals. And with that, meal time truly is meant to be social and interactive. If you had to spoon feed them every time, you wouldn't eat until they are done, and that experience would be disrupted from what would be its natural state.

The Weston A. Price Foundation has some amazing resources on their website for infant nutrition. You can check it out at westonaprice. org. They are big proponents of consuming raw milk. Personally, I don't believe that we need the milk of another species after being weaned off of our own mother's milk. However, I did find raw goat's milk to be highly beneficial and helpful to me to supplement my baby's feeds when I struggled with my breastmilk supply. While there are health benefits to consuming raw milk, I don't find it necessary, especially if you've been able to breastfeed for at least 6–12 months or longer. I bring up Weston Price, because I believe it was their correlation and suggestion that grains not be introduced into a baby's diet until after their molars have first erupted. This is the signal that developmentally they are ready to consume some grains. By grains I mean things like bread, pasta, potatoes, rice, oatmeal, etc. These foods are not as highly nutritious due to the refinement process, and the starches turn into sugar in their bodies. Therefore, it is best to limit these and wait as long as possible before introducing them (if at all).

Lastly, let's discuss allergy concerns. If you have any food sensitivities or allergies, there is a strong possibility that your child has them too. So, it's important to go slowly with what foods you're introducing when, so as to be aware of any potential reactions. If you give too much variety too quickly, it can be difficult to determine what food set off a response. The general rule of thumb is to introduce one food every few days, and watch for reactions. Sometimes allergies take several days or doses to hit a threshold in the body to where the problem becomes apparent. This is why slow and methodical introduction is the way to go.

Truthfully, this topic of food introduction is near and dear to my heart. I could tell you so many stories—here's one of my favorites that illustrates the importance of establishing that groundwork in these beginning days.

I had an experience years ago when my family was apple picking around Labor Day as part of one of my favorite family traditions. I believe it was when Noah was about 10 months old. The place where we go has an amazing farm—there is a petting zoo, playground for the kids, apple picking, a train, jumping pad, and more fun activities. They also have delicious apple cider donuts. I'm not a donut "person," per se, so I might have a bite of one and call it a day. My husband, however, will get a dozen for himself and eat them all within a couple days!

Please don't judge him…HAHA.

So, this particular year, I remember chatting with another mom at the playground when we were there. She had a baby in a stroller that was about 8 months old. We connected over typical baby related topics, especially as the older siblings ran around and played like crazy. It was at that moment that she broke off a piece of an apple cider donut and stuffed it in her baby's mouth stating, "he needs to have the full experience." I was astonished. I don't want to judge. To each their own. I'm just a proponent of educated choices. An 8-month-old would never know the difference or care about a donut if she hadn't made him care. Babies don't care if they have the "full experience" of apple picking. Those small bites set the foundation for a lifetime of cravings for sugar and nutritionally void/toxic foods.

Now, don't get me wrong, all my kids still love sugar. If we asked them if they wanted some zucchini or a cookie for a snack, they would unanimously say "COOKIE!" (Who wouldn't!?) But when first growing accustomed to foods/textures/tastes, there's no reason to begin there. But what about your baby's first birthday??? They need a cake, right? Yes—on my kids 1st birthdays, we did the traditional smash cake thing. It's adorable watching them grab their cake and frosting and smear it all over themselves. It's a rite of passage of sorts. But I made it. It's the concept we addressed earlier, about being able to eat anything you want if you make it yourself. When you make your own food, you have control over the ingredients and therefore have the ability to keep it cleaner and healthier than if you were to buy the exact same thing commercially. There are tons of recipes for applesauce cakes. I made chocolate quinoa cake for at least one of my kids 1st birthdays. I didn't use much, if any, sugar. Why not? They don't know the difference. You generally want their own "smash cake" anyway, so they don't taint the cake being served to guests with their spit and germs. So, it's easy to make your own cake for them using quality ingredients that you can trust.

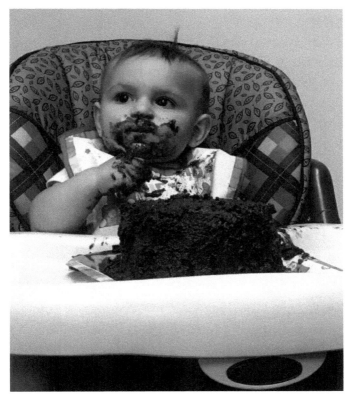

Payton at his first birthday with his homemade chocolate quinoa cake

Here are a few recipes that I would recommend, and of course you can google more. Use search terms like "healthy," "grain free," "gluten free," baby cake recipes.

"Healthy Smash Cake for Baby"
https://www.leahsplate.com/healthy-smash-cake-for-baby/

- 4 ripe bananas (mashed): make sure the bananas are RIPE – this is so important! The bananas are what I use to naturally sweeten the cake.
- 1/2 cup organic unsweetened applesauce: also used to naturally sweeten this cake.
- 3 tbsp. avocado oil OR liquid coconut oil: I really have no preference to using avocado oil or coconut oil as both work really well and are both healthy sources of fat. Please do NOT use canola oil as this is a highly refined inflammatory oil.
- 2 tsp vanilla extract: to give the cake a delicious vanilla flavor.
- 1 tsp baking soda: to help the cake rise while baking.
- 1/4 cup coconut flour: a great grain-free and gluten-free flour substitute and a healthy fat.
- 3/4 cup oat flour: a great gluten-free flour to use and is packed with fiber.
- 1 tsp cinnamon: to give the cake delicious flavor. I love this warming spice.

"Chocolate Quinoa Cake"
https://www.makingthymeforhealth.com/best-ever-chocolate-quinoa-cake-gluten-free/

- 2 cups cooked quinoa*
- 1/3 cup unsweetened almond milk (or preferred milk)
- 4 whole pasture-raised eggs

- 1 teaspoon vanilla extract
- 1/2 cup vegan butter, melted
- 1/4 cup melted coconut oil
- 1 cup organic evaporated cane juice/ or organic white sugar/ or coconut sugar
- 1 cup unsweetened cocoa powder
- 1/2 teaspoon baking soda
- 1 and 1/2 teaspoon baking powder
- 1/2 teaspoon salt

Bottom line, in my opinion, when you're introducing food, think about what we would eat if we weren't tempted by the crap in the stores. Think about what we would consume if we were back to being hunters/gatherers in nature. Think about what our bodies were designed for eating, and feed that to your baby!

9

Baby's Sleep Struggles

Parent sleep—it's like regular sleep, but without the sleep.

I'll admit, it's much easier for me to have the perspectives I will share with you, now that I'm out of the baby stage. But remember, I <u>was</u> where you are. Three times. I lost sleep, and in some ways those early months are just a blur. But we women are strong as hell and can get through it!!! So, let's talk about sleep. I want to dispel a few myths right off the bat.

1. Adding cereal to your baby's bottle will help them sleep longer without waking.
2. Your baby should be sleeping through the night by the time they are 3 months old.
3. You should never sleep with your baby in your bed.
4. You should never nurse your baby to sleep.
5. You will need to let your baby self soothe.

I'd like to go through these myths one by one. And, I remind you, as I have throughout the book so far, that I am not here to judge anyone's parenting style or decisions. I am only here to provide an alternate perspective that I've used, and feel is a good approach. However, these methods don't work for everyone, and I understand that. The bottom line is to do what works best for you and your family while keeping everyone healthy and sane!

ADDING CEREAL TO THE BABY'S BOTTLE TO KEEP THEM ASLEEP LONGER

This is one of the most outdated pieces of advice I have ever heard. I'm weird with a lot of my methods, but even this isn't recommended by the World Health Organization. Solids are not advisable until at least 6 months of age, and it is a choking hazard to add solids to a bottle. Additionally, as we discussed in the last chapter, rice cereal offers little to no nutritional value whatsoever and should not be considered in the realm of "first foods" to feed your child anyway.

SLEEPING THROUGH THE NIGHT

The notion that your baby should be sleeping through the night at a specific age is ridiculous. I know one of the most common questions you're asked about your infant in the first year of life is, "so, how does he/she sleep? —Sleeping through the night yet?" I came to hate this question. My answer was always a "NO!"—and it made me feel bad. Like I was doing something wrong. The mom guilt and perceived judgement from those simple words and questions were intense. So, I encourage you to let it go!! Every baby, just like every adult is different. We all have different cycles, rhythms, and a developmental pace at which milestones are reached. Sleep is one of those developmental stages. Of course if a baby is full, they will sleep longer and better than if they are hungry. However, assuming your child is getting what they need nutritionally through breastmilk or formula, the amount isn't going to influence their sleep schedule. Additionally, frequent waking is protective against SIDS! So, we can change our perspective to that of gratitude for our interrupted sleep!

You may get lucky and have an excellent sleeper that slept through the night by 3–4 weeks old. (If you're in this camp, consider this a "congratulations" from me, but I won't be talking to you until the end of this chapter!—(just kidding, kind of). You may get some that don't "sleep through the night" until they are over 1 year old (like mine!) Then there are babies that fall everywhere in between. And guess what? They are all normal! If they are fed, comforted, loved, growing, peeing, pooping, and getting stronger—they will find their groove with sleep at some point. The other tricks I utilized whenever possible were remedies such as homeopathy, flower essences, essential oils, and chiropractic/energy work from myself and colleagues.

CO-SLEEPING

This topic usually gets heated. Some are strongly against the practice of sleeping with your baby, while others wouldn't have a child without doing so. What I can tell you is that your opinion of any practice surrounding child-rearing changes when you become a parent. I never thought I'd have my kids in my bed. Maybe once in awhile because of a bad dream when they were older—but how things change. And that's ok! Remember, you do what works best for you and your family. I just want to throw out a few statistics about co-sleeping so that if you're having a hard time like I did, you know it's not a bad solution. In fact, it's the most natural solution to get yourself and your child better, more quality sleep.

First off, I'd like to remind you that we are a part of the animal kingdom. We are physiologically no different that our evolutionary ancestors. Our only difference is our cultural habitats. If we were still living in caveman days, would our children sleep in a different cave? Or a separate tree far away from us? Absolutely not. It would be the safest and easiest to keep your infant close by.

Here are the following benefits that come from sleeping with your baby: more regular and stable respiration, temperature and heartbeat, lowered incidence of SIDS, lowered anxiety of separation for baby and mom, better chance of good milk supply, increased bonding, and comfort. It is the most natural thing in the world that somehow has become weird or unsafe. Assuming that you're not abusing alcohol or drugs, you are completely safe to have your baby sleep in your bed. You have a 6th sense about you. You will intuitively know your child is there and not roll over them. You obviously won't smother them with blankets. But snuggling with your baby is the most precious moment you can cherish. Plus, it makes it easier on you to respond to their needs in the middle of the night without getting insanely sleep deprived yourself. This actually allows for better sleep for you too!

There are different methods of co-sleeping. You can have your baby straight up in your bed, or you can invest in what's called a "co-sleeper." This is kind of like an extension of your bed, so it allows you to be close to your child, but also provides you space and keeps you comfortable so that you can move more freely. This is kind of the best of both worlds in a sense. I never had one. I didn't know any of this with my first child. I wish I had! I would say looking back, I slept with my babies until they were about 6 months old, and then I transitioned them to their own crib. At that point they would start the night there, and upon their first wake, finish the night with us. This is what worked for me. I don't know what will work for you. You will find your groove. I'm here to tell you that it is OKAY to sleep with your baby. Many more parents do it than you know or think would. It's normal, it's natural, and it's healthy.

NURSING TO SLEEP

I'll come out and admit this freely – I ALWAYS nursed my babies to sleep, against all the mainstream advice. I heard it all. "You don't want to become a human pacifier." "You'll never get them off of you doing that." "You're teaching them bad habits." Once again, I know plenty of women who have done it, and felt the same way that I did. Like a failure. Like you're doing something wrong. There is ONE wrong ways to treat a child–abuse! Comfort nursing your child to sleep is not wrong. Sometimes we do what is easiest to get us through the tough times. In my world, boobs were magic. Even though I didn't produce a lot of milk, my boys were deeply comforted by nursing and that was the best gift I feel I ever gave them.

There are plenty of methods that teach you to have your baby nurse until they are almost asleep, and then put them down groggy, but awake so that they fall asleep on their own and aren't "dependent" on you for falling asleep. These methods never worked for me, but I know others who swear by them. Either way, it is okay and not harmful to nurse to sleep. I promise you they will not go to college unable to sleep without your breast.

"SELF-SOOTHING"

Self-soothing is also known as the "cry it out" method of sleep training. I never could let my kids cry themselves to sleep. It went against every ounce of my being as a mother, and I couldn't do it. Again, if we were in caveman days, if we let our child cry until they fell asleep, they would be eaten by a predator before they had the chance to do so! Luckily in our modern day society, that is not a risk. But when you begin the process of letting your child cry without your response to their needs, I feel it breaks the relationship and trust. This little being who has depended on you for so much suddenly doesn't see you when they cry. I've often read suggestions in parenting books that literally hurts my heart. Suggestions such as "be ready to change the bed. Some babies scream so hard that they are sick, so put a spare sheet next to the bed…Try to be efficient and calm as you change the sheet, and do half at a time so you don't need to lift your baby out. Don't speak to your baby, and be as quick as you can so that you don't get their hopes up allowing him to think that he's going to be cuddled and fed."

This breaks my heart to hear that this kind of cruel and neglectful behavior is being passed off as advice for new mothers. I understand that there comes a point when you have to teach your baby to sleep. But there are plenty of ways to do it that do not involve listening to your baby scream for an hour. Have you every cried yourself to sleep? After an argument with your spouse? Or after losing a loved one? Or after another traumatic event? How did it feel? Did you wake up feeling refreshed the next morning? Or sad, disconnected, and depleted? Now imagine this growing little being that has no control over anything in his/her new world.

Cortisol is the stress hormone that mammals produce in response to a threat, real or perceived. A study was done measuring the cortisol levels of mom and baby during sleep training. The results? Night 1 – Baby was stressed and crying, and mom was stressed because the baby was crying, so both had elevated levels of cortisol. Night 2 – the same as night 1. Night 3 – baby didn't cry. Mom's stress and cortisol went down assuming he/she had learned to self-soothe. But in reality, the baby's cortisol levels were higher than the other nights when they'd been crying. The baby never stopped being stressed; they just learned that their mother wouldn't respond, so they didn't cry. This can actually disrupt their body's ability to achieve a level of deep sleep, potentially lead to insecure attachments, and affect moral and psychosocial development. Here is the link to the study https://pubmed.ncbi.nlm.nih.gov/21945361/.

Now, for the record, I also know plenty of people who have chosen to sleep train their children in this way, and there appears to be no long term damage from it at all. If you google it, you'll find plenty of research proving that this method has no adverse effects on baby's development. But, if you're like me, looking for another way, know that there is one. You don't need to feel forced to let your baby "cry it out" if you don't want to. I especially wouldn't recommend it before a year, and never before 6–9 months. You want to at the very least establish a strong relationship of trust first. I never said my way was easy, but I do believe it is worth it. I've also included more book references in the resources section for you to check out or google with regard to other non-cry-it-out sleep training methods.

I also recently had a patient tell me that simply putting her baby on a different schedule was incredibly impactful for the baby, and quite frankly her sleep as well! Sometimes putting them down a little earlier or later may resonate better with their body and system, and make all the difference in the world. And what worked for the first few months may not work later on. Illness, teething, developmental changes, and more can affect the quality of your baby's sleep. Motherhood, just like life, is about adapting. Roll with the changes, and do the best you can!

There are homeopathic remedies that can be incredibly powerful to balance sleep, stress, teething pain, and irritability in your baby. Additionally, chiropractic care is paramount to removing the blockages in the nervous system to aid in better sleep. I have several patients where after I treated their babies, they would call and tell me that they slept for the longest chunk of time that they had up until that point. I don't always assume miracles like this will occur, but they have happened. When we address the chemical, emotional, and structural reasons for sleep imbalances, the results can be astounding!

10

Baby's Immune System

The best and most efficient pharmacy is within your own system
-Robert C. Peahle

Welcome to the part of the book where you'll learn everything you need to know about how to keep your child truly healthy— even through all the immune and health challenges that he/she may face. Now, this chapter is not all related to the immune system, or illness. However, a lot of it is, and it will offer some suggestions that you may not have heard of before. As a holistic physician, I choose to heal and treat most ailments with non-pharmacological methods. In fact, my boys have never had an antibiotic or any prescription in their whole lives, and they are 10, 7, and 5 years old. This is not to say they haven't been sick. Things happen. Life happens. Getting sick is a normal and natural part of immune building. If we aren't exposed to any germs, our immune systems fail to develop and when finally challenged with a virus or bacteria, our body would not know how to react and we would be more sick as a result. (Extreme isolation/lockdown with Covid-19 has definitely been an immune challenge for many!) That said, babies have their immune system built and started during birth and nursing as discussed previously. Vaginal birth begins the microbiome foundation. (Microbiome is a term that refers to the diversity of probiotic organisms that are meant to live in the gut). This first inoculation of bacteria is critical to a healthy microbiome, and many babies these days are robbed of that due to the increasing number of cesarean births. I previously shared my suggestion to mitigate this. This is the normal process that would have happened with a vaginal birth, so attempting to recreate it as best as possible is worth the shot!

The second way your baby begins building his/her immune system and microbiome is through breastfeeding. You have normal bacteria living on your skin to maintain your health, and through a symbiotic relationship, they help keep other unwanted bugs out. Every time your baby latches, or even simply cuddles skin-to-skin, they are absorbing more bacteria to add to their bodies for development. So, even if breastfeeding wasn't an option for you, skin-to-skin contact is a fantastic way to transfer some of these normal "bugs" to your baby.

The immune system and general health are incredibly important to much of what will be discussed here. I wouldn't recommend the following suggestions if they haven't been powerfully effective in my own kids, or patients I've treated. Or both. ☺ I'll go through these topics one at a time. I feel that it is a pretty comprehensive list of what most parents will experience in the first 1-2 years of their children's lives, and may want guidance on. If there is something that you don't see on this list that you'd like support with, my information is at the end of the book under resources. I am happy to be a source of support for you even after you've finished reading!

COLIC/SPIT UP ISSUES

Your baby's digestive system is still new and underdeveloped. So, things like gas and spitting up can be very common things to experience. However, they aren't normal. If your baby is crying clearly from gassiness or spits up a large amount frequently, there are reasons for it. The first that I find most often is related to food allergies/sensitivities. As I said, your baby's digestive tract is immature—meaning that the "tight junctions" in the small intestine have not formed yet. Therefore, all proteins that your baby ingests can easily go straight into the bloodstream because they don't have the protection to prevent it. I've seen time and time again simply getting a child on a different formula, or simply taking something out of the mother's diet if she's nursing, can be a literal night and day difference in their health and comfort. The most common allergens I find in practice are dairy (cow's milk), soy, and gluten. There are others, but if we are just guessing, these are a good start. Take these out of your diet if you're exclusively breastfeeding, or check the ingredients of your formula. Dairy comes in the form of "casein" frequently when you're reading labels.

Homeopathic remedies can be very effective and powerful, but I always like to assess a child first before suggesting a remedy. I would almost always address the root cause, especially if it's as simple as removing one food, because without that you'll be constantly reinjuring the system without knowing it.

Spitting up can be a tricky one. Some spit up is normal as your baby begins to figure out how to regulate feedings. During this time, their nervous system also develops the esophageal sphincter tone and function to keep food in the stomach. This just takes time to normalize as baby grows. My babies rarely spit up a lot unless we overfed them.

I love working on babies in my office to check the integrity of their nervous system and organ structure and function. I frequently find abdominal spasms, hiatal hernias, and other imbalances in baby's guts. And most of the time, these issues are resolved in 1-2 treatments. The key is acting fast. When working with pregnant women, to encourage them to come in quickly after birth to rebalance their own body, I offer a free treatment to their baby at that first postpartum visit because I recognize the importance of chiropractic and kinesiological care on infants. Therefore, I HIGHLY recommend getting your baby evaluated as early as possible by an Applied Kinesiology chiropractic physician, or at least a pediatric chiropractor.

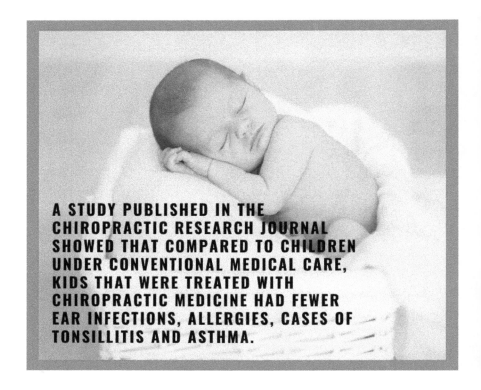

A STUDY PUBLISHED IN THE CHIROPRACTIC RESEARCH JOURNAL SHOWED THAT COMPARED TO CHILDREN UNDER CONVENTIONAL MEDICAL CARE, KIDS THAT WERE TREATED WITH CHIROPRACTIC MEDICINE HAD FEWER EAR INFECTIONS, ALLERGIES, CASES OF TONSILLITIS AND ASTHMA.

BABY ACNE

Baby acne is relatively normal due to the influx of hormonal exchange between the mother and the baby during birth and breastfeeding. Rarely is it a problem, and it generally resolves on its own within a few weeks. I found that applying breastmilk to any acne spots topically can help them heal faster!

CRADLE CAP

All my kids had some level of cradle cap as babies. It's usually advisable to leave it alone and let it heal and dissipate naturally. However, this can take some time, and depending on the severity, can be quite unsightly and irritating. I believe that one can gently and safely comb through it. Coconut oil helps to loosen it up a bit to allow for increased ease of removal. Remember, if you choose to do this, be <u>very</u> gentle, especially around the baby's soft spot, and be aware of your baby's disposition in the process. If he/she appears distressed as a result, stop immediately and leave the area alone.

DIAPER RASH AND OTHER SKIN IRRITATIONS

Frequent diaper changes help to alleviate rashes in baby's nether-regions. That said, sometimes it happens. I always recommend coconut oil as it's the most natural, and has antiviral, antifungal and antibacterial properties. It's perfect for topical application to most skin eruptions including eczema. Other than coconut oil, Weleda is a brand of cream I've used before that I completely support. The active ingredients in it are zinc, beeswax, calendula, and natural oils. Natural and healing. I'll be honest—I've even used it on myself for chafing or simple heat rash, and it usually takes care of it within a day or two. What hasn't cleared up with coconut oil and breastmilk topically has been helped by this Weleda Diaper cream!

As for other rashes like eczema are concerned, I've seen many kids in my practice with this ailment—99% of the time it is an allergy. Food is one of the first things I look into—and if breast-feeding, it can absolutely be something mom is eating causing the reaction in the baby. I NEVER recommend topically utilizing steroid creams. Inevitably, steroid creams in such small humans disrupt adrenal gland function, and over time frequently lead to the development of asthma in those children later in life. So, if your child suffers from skin rashes, first look to the diet. Wheat (gluten), dairy, corn, soy, citrus, sugar, and nuts tend to be the most common culprits in my experience. But everyone is different. I've seen some kids even sensitive to green beans—so, it's important to consult with a holistic care provider to determine the root cause of the rash, instead of suppressing it. When you artificially suppress a symptom, the body will generally find another way of expressing its "dis-ease," and at that point, I find the secondary method it chooses to communicate that imbalance will be more severe than the first.

Our son Luke was a little over a year old when he started having a rash around his mouth and chin. We tried our own treatments for a couple months, and it kept getting worse. We thought that it was due to food allergies, so we decided to take him to an allergist to get help figuring it out. When we took him, the doctor treated him for impetigo and eczema. She said it was so bad that he needed to take oral antibiotics, a topical steroid, and Benadryl to keep him out of the hospital. We followed this doctor's treatment the first time loosely because it felt like a lot of medicine to put in a 1 1/2 year old body all at once. The rash got better with the treatment, but it came back almost 2 days after the treatment was over. The doctor said to do the same treatment exactly as she prescribed, and to give him Benadryl indefinitely. We followed it, and the rash came back even though we continued with the Benadryl. The allergist said the eczema will never go away and has nothing to do with food allergies. We didn't believe her, and we decided it was time to go elsewhere. Luke's primary care physician ordered an allergy blood test, but nothing significant showed up on that.

In addition to seeing several natural providers for probiotics and immune boosting supplements, we started doing our own elimination diet because we just knew Luke's rash had something to do with food. While adding more foods into his diet, it became apparent that we wanted help figuring out what foods were good and what ones were not, so we saw Dr. Christy Matusiak. We brought a bagful of foods we were questioning as problematic, and she did muscle testing to give us some clarity. She also gave Luke adjustments, an essential oil blend, and a homeopathic spray.

Luke's rash got significantly better over the months since we stopped following the allergist's advice and reached out to others, but it would still occasionally return. Luke's face was the clearest when we had him on a diet closely related to the Autoimmune Protocol Diet, but that was not sustainable for our family. We have recently begun NAET treatment, and Luke's diet has been expanding and his rash is barely noticeable most days. It has never become infected since we stopped following the allergists' advice. We knew there was something deeper going on in Luke's body, and that the skin was just the display of it. Luke also knew what treatments were good for his body, and what ones were not. It was a huge challenge to get him to take the prescriptions from the allergist, yet he has never refused any probiotics, cod liver oil, vitamins, elderberry, astragalus root, etc. We are so grateful for all the practitioners who have helped us on this journey.
-Kristin R.

BATHING SOAPS/LOTIONS

I get very picky about what I choose to put on my own skin and my children's. My rule of thumb, is that if you couldn't or wouldn't eat it, don't put it on your skin. The skin is the largest organ of the body and is highly absorptive. The body takes in anything topical through the pores, and it goes straight into the bloodstream. This is not great if you read some of the labels of commercial soaps, lotions, and sunscreens marketed for newborns and infants! I understand no one would want to eat soap, but I'm just asking you to read the ingredient list of topical products you consider using, just as you would something you would eat. If you recognize everything, it's likely a good product. If not? Run! For instance, let's compare these two products marketed for baby hygiene.

Frequently marketed name brand for baby soap:

Water*, Cocamidopropyl Betaine*, Decyl Glucoside, Sodium Cocoyl Isethionate*, Lauryl Glucoside*, PEG-80 Sorbitan Laurate, Glycerin*, Citric Acid*, Sodium Benzoate, PEG-150 Distearate, Sodium Methyl Cocoyl Taurate*, Fragrance [Benzyl Acetate, Ionone Beta, Methyl Ionones, Peach Pure, Phenyl Ethyl Alcohol, Tropional], Polyquaternium-10, Disodium EDTA.

*Naturally derived ingredient

Weleda baby brand:

Water (aqua), coco-glucoside, prunus amygdalus dulcis (sweet almond) oil, alcohol, disodium cocoyl glutamate, sesamum indicum (sesame) seed oil, glycerin, carrageenan, sodium cocoyl glutamate, calendula officinalis flower extract, xanthan gum, lactic acid, fragrance (parfum)*, limonene*, linalool*.

*From natural essential oils.

Which ingredients do you recognize more of and could feasibly recreate the recipe if forced to? Just like with food, we can't always make EVERYTHING ourselves—but when reading labels, if you COULD make it yourself, then it's likely that it's a healthier product than if you had no idea what half of the ingredients were.

The last thing I want to mention here under the topic of skin health is sunscreen. Of course we do not want our baby getting sunburned! At the same time, most conventional sunscreens have incredibly toxic ingredients that I'd never recommend you put on your child. As far as sun protection goes, I find it beneficial for the purposes of vitamin D production to let your baby get some natural un-interrupted sun exposure. Their skin is obviously much more sensitive than an adult, so 10-15 minutes in direct summer sunlight is likely the most I'd do before seeking shade for him/her. Otherwise, Badger is one of the best brands I have found for nontoxic sunblock. Its active ingredient is zinc oxide, and inactive ingredients include sunflower oil, beeswax, vitamin E, calendula, and chamomile. There is even a special "baby" version! But there are many more quality products out there. That example is one of many. My point is to simply begin being an educated consumer. Look up things you don't know or don't understand. My goal is to teach you to fish for yourself—not just feed you all the fish. If that were the case, this book would be never ending, and you'd get tired of me!

BLOCKED TEAR DUCTS

This is another common ailment in newborns that, thankfully, none of my babies had. However, I have patients that have told me their babies had developed conjunctivitis within the first few weeks of birth due to a blocked tear duct that quickly escalated. In a clogged tear duct, your baby's eyelid may become swollen and red, like a sty. Warm, clean washcloths are the first easy defense against this, and can be very helpful. But I find that it's sometimes not enough. My best solution to this: Breastmilk drops in/around their eye. Even if you put it on their closed eye while your baby is sleeping, when he/she opens their eyes, there will be a small amount of milk that will get into the eye and begin working to heal the inflammation. Breastmilk is magic—did you know that every drop of breastmilk has 1-5 MILLION white blood cells to help fight infections? That's just in one drop!! I use breastmilk for eye infections, ear infections, rashes, and even scrapes and contusions when they get older. It's easy and portable anywhere! When they finally wean, and breastmilk isn't as easily accessible anymore, coconut oil is my favorite antibacterial/antiviral topical agent.

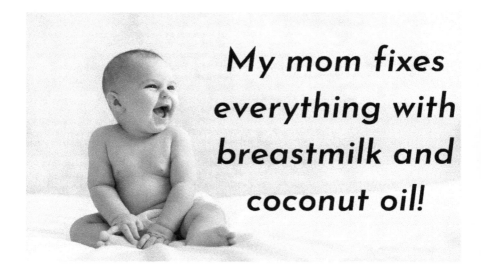

My mom fixes everything with breastmilk and coconut oil!

There are other homeopathic eye drops that I recommend for adults and older children for eye irritation and infections, but I generally haven't found them necessary for infants. Breastmilk will do the job within a few days. Similasan drops are my other suggestion if the above takes longer than 3 days to see progress. Please reference the resources in the back of the book to learn more about dosing homeopathy.

FEVERS

Uh oh. Your baby has a fever. What do you do? Mainstream suggestions say alternate baby Tylenol and Advil to reduce it. I want to communicate something really important to you here—FEVERS ARE A GOOD THING. They indicate that the body is fighting off a foreign invader. It means the child is sick. But it doesn't mean you have to panic. Fevers up to 104 degrees Fahrenheit are acceptable. They can absolutely be scary—and I'm not saying to do nothing—but you can respect the body's process and support it as it works through the immune challenge. When we suppress a fever, we take away the ability of a higher temperature to kill the virus or bacteria. Therefore, it's a strong likelihood that the illness will last longer as a result of reducing fever. We trade healing for short term comfort. There are two homeopathic remedies I like to use and recommend when a child has a fever. Ferrum Phosphoricum for a low-grade fever and nonspecific symptoms, or Belladonna for an acute red hot kind of high fever. I suggest using 30C potency for both. If you're not familiar with homeopathy, allow me to explain:

Homeopathy is based on the principle that like cures like. So, for example, if you were bit by a snake that released venom into your system, the philosophy of homeopathy would go like this – take a drop of that snake venom. And dilute it in 10 ml of water. Then, take a drop of that solution, and dilute it again. Then, take a drop of that dilution, and dilute it again—and again—and again. That process is repeated until there is no detectable amount of the original substance present. What you're left with is an energetic imprint and the frequency of the offending issue. When introduced to the body in that dilution, the body can then take it and mount an immune response to fight it. Where other methods of care alleviate symptoms by suppression, homeopathy allows the body to do what it was meant to do—fight naturally.

If you'd like to learn more about homeopathy and get a guide of what remedies are best in given situations, I frequently recommend patients get the book: *Homeopathic Self-Care,* by Robert Ullman, ND and Judyth Reichenberg-Ullman, ND, to add to their health resource library. It's not always 100% helpful, but it's a completely safe method to utilize when something is concerning with your or your child's health. Antibiotics, and other Western approaches will still be there and available if they are absolutely necessary, and sometimes they are. But, more often than not—they aren't required, and can cause more harm than good.

For instance, even in mainstream medicine, gut health is incredibly important. Frequent antibiotic regimens disrupt the proper flora balance in the large intestine, and can cause constipation, diarrhea, skin rashes, mental/emotional disturbances, and much more. Research is continually showing that the appropriate bacterial balance in the gut is one of the most critical components of health. Besides antibiotics, Tylenol has been studied for its potential carcinogenic (cancer causing) effects. While a lot of these products can save lives in a necessary emergency, they should not be overused—especially when there are many safer alternatives available.

Aside from homeopathy, there is one other magical trick I swear by with fever. It's called the wet-sock treatment. It sounds awful, but I promise it isn't as bad as it sounds. You need 2 pairs of socks—one pair of thin, cotton socks, and another set of thick, warm, wool socks. Begin by wetting the thin pair with cold water. Wring them out so they aren't dripping and just damp, and place them in the freezer for about 10-15 minutes. Place the cold socks on your child's feet before they go to sleep for the night. Then cover them with the thick, warm, dry socks. This contrast of temperatures, literally pulls the fever out of the body overnight and stimulates the immune system to heal.

Early on raising kids I believed in "Motrinning" a fever to death, antibiotics, and whatever was a quick fix. Over time too many antibiotics, and poor eating led me to find a more holistic approach to my kids' health to help stomach issues, recurring ear infections, and severe cases of croup that didn't go away with age, and mood swings. I met Dr. Matusiak when my kids were 10, 8, and 5. Whenever sick, my kids were always totally up for going to "that doctor's office." They always seemed to feel better after. They also were good at abiding by the suggestions, because they always seemed to help quickly.

I had to laugh when my middle son was eager to try her seemingly crazy (not to mention miserable sounding) "frozen sock trick" suggestion to help his fever, when he came down with pretty severe flu symptoms. I was shivering as I reached my hand in the large bowl of ice water to wring out the socks I drenched. I pushed the socks onto his feet, and rolled up his legs. He was such a trooper and said it oddly felt amazing. We then covered it with dry socks and laid a towel on his sheets to help keep the bed dry. He fell asleep and when he woke up a couple of hours later, the socks were bone dry and his fever was gone. It literally pulled it out of him.

All of my kids have sworn by this, and yes, I had to succumb to their pressure to try when I was sick and have to attest it was amazing and fascinating how it worked. Most times, the kids fevers never came back at all, or if so, mildly and we did it again. I had to laugh again, when my oldest informed me he did this on his own when he was miserable and sick living in his fraternity house in college. I must tell you it is worth the effort and temporary misery! -Cheri W.

COLDS/FLUS

Once again, homeopathy is my go-to with these sorts of issues. When your baby falls sick, assuming you're still nursing, the best thing you can do is to continue snuggling and nursing that cherub as often and as long as they want. They need the comfort and warmth of you, their caregiver and first love. The breastmilk obviously contains all the antibodies and immune support they will need to overcome the illness. If this is no longer enough, and/or your baby is older, oscilliococcinum is a fantastic flu aid homeopathic remedy. For children under 2 years old, I don't recommend giving an entire tube – but you can use 1/4 - 1/2 a tube to support flu. For colds, there are tons of remedies available depending on the specific complaint. (Allium Cepa, Pulsatilla, Hepar Sulpharis, Antimonium tartaricum...and much more!) This is not a book about homeopathy, which is why I suggest the book I referenced earlier. But I firmly believe that this is a better system than over the counter drugs to suppress symptoms. Homeopathy is the easiest to give in babies before they are eating solid foods, where you can at that point, sneak liquid or powdered vitamins into applesauce. But when they are still infants, homeopathy works like a charm—you can put the pellets directly into the baby's mouth or dissolve them in a bottle.

TEETHING

The classic teething remedy is Chamomilla 30C. Hyland's has a good blend of homeopathy that includes Chamomilla in its complex to reduce and manage teething pain, discomfort, and general fussiness. There have been times where my kids were teething and they were MISERABLE— I couldn't put them down for even a few minutes without tears—1-2 doses of the right remedy allowed them to sleep alone for hours! It can literally be magic, without any toxic side effects!

Some friends of mine swear by Amber teething necklaces. I don't have personal experience with these, but don't find them harmful. It's worth a shot, as long as you're mindful and careful about them as a choking hazard.

EAR INFECTIONS

In my experience, ear infections in young ones are 99% viral, and children are vulnerable to getting them when they have a dairy sensitivity. It's so common, and even if one is not dairy sensitive, cow's milk products tend to be very pro-inflammatory and create a lot of excess mucus. It's always a good idea to eliminate cow's milk from baby's diet, or your diet if breastfeeding during illness. And most chiropractors are highly skilled in eliminating ear pain in childhood ear infections through adjustments, muscle work, and nutrition therapy. Not all chiropractors are created equal, of course— I'll offer a list of chiropractic websites at the end of the book as resources, so you can make a good decision with the type of doctor you choose to work with.

VACCINES

Before you freak out during this section, please know that I am NOT anti-vaccination. I am pro-choice of which vaccinations one chooses to give their child, and on what schedule. It's a fact that since I was a child, the number of vaccines that a child is expected to receive by the time they are 18 years old has more than TRIPLED. Why is that? And why should you care?

These immunizations do not come without risk. Any medical procedure that carries with it any risk, requires informed consent. That means your medical provider should be able to provide you with the benefits, risks, and alternatives of their recommended intervention. This is rarely, if ever, done with regard to routine vaccinations. I encourage you to look up a real package insert from the pharmaceutical company to see for yourself the potential risks, side effects, and ingredients in a standard dose. You'll be surprised.

Now, I get it. We don't want our kids getting sick—especially if we know that we could prevent them from getting an illness in the first place!!! So my method of assessment is that of risk/benefit analysis. If a particular illness is incredibly dangerous and deadly, and the vaccination has been around for a long time without significantly reported adverse reactions, then that would be one to highly consider giving to your child. On the other hand, if an illness is something you, yourself, had as a child, for all intents and purposes rarely poses complications, and is relatively new to the CDC recommended schedule, that would be one on my list to consider refusing. This should not be an all-or-nothing topic. For instance, Hepatitis B vaccination is required at birth—WHY? Hep B is transmitted via blood and via sexual contact. If the mother is Hepatitis B negative, there is literally no risk of the infant contracting this illness, unless they require a blood transfusion where blood could be contaminated. So what's the reasoning behind this? In case the mother was promiscuous during the pregnancy and could have contracted Hep B without being detected on initial pre-natal bloodwork, it's recommended all infants are immunized on day one of life. As if birth isn't traumatic enough, we think it's a good idea to inject aluminum and formaldehyde into their bloodstream before their body is capable of detoxifying yet. I have heard the argument that we want the child to be prepared and protected for when they become sexually active. That's a conversation for 12 years down the road—not on day one of his/her life. Boosters are generally required anyway, so why start with it as a newborn?!

I'm not recommending any schedule, or refusal of any specific vaccines here. I just want to encourage you to think critically. *The Vaccine Book,* by Dr. Robert W. Sears, MD, FAAP, is an excellent resource—and a completely neutral one, where you can read the unbiased facts about each disease/immunization so you can truly make an informed decision on how to proceed with your child's schedule. As a general rule, I suggest waiting as long as possible to introduce these toxins into your baby's bloodstream, so as to give them the time to build the resiliency and capacity to handle the shots, with the ability to break down the chemicals properly. If/when those times come, there is a protocol and homeopathic remedy I recommend to my patients to give to their children prior to and immediately following immunizations to help their bodies handle it better.

TO CIRCUMCISE OR NOT TO CIRCUMCISE

If you have a little girl, you can thankfully skip through this section. However, with baby boys, the inevitable question comes up before or shortly after birth—are you going to have him circumcised? This is an incredibly personal decision. There are many religious traditions and cultural reasons to have it performed. However, there are no medical reasons for which doctors currently recommend it. In the past, it was declared to be cleaner and less likely to get infections when circumcised.

This information has since been shown to be untrue. The foreskin is the natural protection to keep the penis safe from feces and other contaminants. Simple hygiene is all that needs to be employed here. But this is a highly debated topic, and I highly encourage you to look into the information for yourself to make the best decision for your child. If you choose to have it done, homeopathic Arnica Montana 30C would be indicated to help him recover from the trauma quickly—along with lots of snuggles and nursing.

11

Baby's Physical and Neurological Development

Play gives children a chance to practice what they are learning.
-Fred Rogers

Up until now, we've discussed all the ways to keep yourself healthy and sane, as well as how to encourage your baby's healthy growth. We bring our kids to the pediatrician to check in on their physical growth regularly. But how can we ensure they are on the right track, without blockages to their development? Frequently, I find pediatric appointments are great when things are going well, but lack direction when something isn't right. Wouldn't it be nice to have the knowledge ahead of time to be able to properly ensure your child's healthy development to reduce the chances of developmental setbacks?! That's exactly what I'm going to address here!

There are several stages that babies go through as they grow and mature. From the time they are in utero, to about 16 weeks, your baby's movements are fish-like and reflexive in nature. Their motions and movements are disconnected, and there is no purposeful mobility. During this stage, the most important thing you can do to encourage your child's progress is tummy time. It is through tummy time that their neck strength is created, developing the proper curvature of their spine. Additionally, it is through this "exercise," that they simply stimulate strength and growth in their muscles and nervous system. Now, I understand, most babies hate tummy time! I'm not saying you need to leave them in that position for hours. If they tolerate it well, great! The more the better. But if they are not a fan, then even just a few minutes several times per day is beneficial. Whenever you have to put them down to use the restroom, answer the phone, get dressed/ shower, or cook dinner, just put them on their belly. Babies are just like adults in that, when we are challenged, we become resourceful. Allow them that opportunity to discover their own body and mechanics to create that resourcefulness. Another hint—in the newborn stage, your baby can do tummy time on your chest. It's a beautiful connecting moment, but also encourages their developing muscles!

The next stage is from 16 weeks until about 6 months of age. This phase is where the baby is in a homolateral pattern. This means that each side of the child's body works independently and eyes/ears therefore are not "yoked" to function together yet. At this point they will not be able to locate sound because there is no functioning depth perception. During the latter part of this stage of development, your baby will begin sitting up, and rolling over. Usually they roll over from their stomach to their back before going from their back to their stomach. Generally, your baby will not have the strength to comfortably and reliably sit on their own until 6 to 8 months old. Prior to that time, it can be tempting to utilize a Bumbo baby seat. This is a little device (see picture below) that positions your child's legs and pelvis in such a way that it allows them to sit up unassisted without worry about them falling over. I highly do NOT recommend using these chairs. As your child is growing and developing strength, it is critical that their own muscles learn what to do. Think of it like this. Let's say you have a back injury. In order to cope with your activities of daily life, you choose to wear a back brace. Those can be helpful in the short term to reduce pain and allow support while you heal. However, that brace acts as an artificial muscle doing what your own body should be able to do. Over time of using it, your muscles get the message that they no longer need to function so they literally shut "off" neurologically. This then causes more weaknesses and imbalances in your structure. The same logic applies behind these baby seats. Your child needs to learn how to sit up on his/her own in their own time and way. Depriving them of this challenge and stage of development out of our own convenience is just not right for their body in the long run. The bottom line is to remember that their freedom of motion should be preserved at all costs for proper development of nervous system function. This also means limiting the usage of playpens and carrying baskets. Tummy time is still the best way for this strength and development to occur.

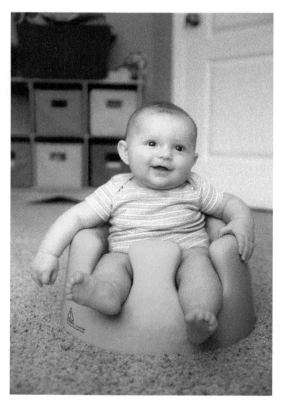

Bumbo seat

Another important concept regarding proper stimulation in these early stages is how we feed our baby. When we breastfeed, nature takes care of this for us as we have to feed from both sides. So during feeds, one eye/arm takes turns being restricted creating balance. If we only bottle feed, we have a tendency to keep the same position/side to feed the child and this prevents them from achieving adequate stimulation from one side, creating slowed and disrupted bilateral development. Therefore, whenever bottle feeding, I highly suggest switching sides/ positions so your baby is not left with one side stronger than the other.

As they grow, around 6 months of age through 1 year, they reach contralateral crawl phase. This is the point where your baby will begin to learn to crawl and develop the coordination of right and left sides together. I can't stress this enough: IT IS IMPORTANT THAT YOUR CHILD CRAWLS. I don't mean army-crawling. I'm talking about hands and knees, alternating right arm with left knee and vice versa – <u>CRAWLING</u>. I know several children whose parents say that their kids never crawled, and just went straight to walking after "scooting" or army-crawling. Skipping this important step can be disadvantageous to their body as they continue to grow. Your child should be relatively proficient at cross-crawl bilateral activity before becoming biped. Frequently as a chiropractor, I address retained primitive reflexes or other patterns that children didn't outgrow as they got older. I have seen kids, who simply don't walk correctly in a proper neurological gait, struggle with athletics in high school. Their muscles don't fire in the appropriate patterns, and this can lead to injuries and reduced performance as a result. This is another reason I always recommend getting kids evaluated by a quality chiropractic physician to correct these imbalances or stuck patterns as early as possible. How early, you ask? I treated my own kids within hours or days of their births. The earlier and more frequent you can have them treated, the better. Birth trauma is real and the quicker we can address and reduce that nerve interference, the less opportunity their body has to develop compensations and layers of dysfunction. That said, if your child begins crawling on their stomach in a scooting-pattern, this isn't necessarily a bad sign. You just want to observe symmetry and gently encourage hands/knees position to create more of a crawling pattern. If he/she prefers spinning to one side, or nurses only on one side, or clearly utilizes one arm/leg more so than the other side, get him/her checked out. My oldest was my earliest crawler (6.5 months) and walker (10 months). I observed him on his tummy for months, before around 5 months old he began bridging up on his hands and knees and rocking back and forth. This is normal, albeit early, progression. Although he was on the early side, early does not always mean better!

If your child isn't crawling by 8 months that doesn't necessarily mean that something is wrong. Every child is on their own timeline of development and achieving milestones. I'm a firm believer in respecting each child's journey and letting them do the leading. We can encourage them, but not force them to do something they aren't ready for. Like I said, my kids were all different! Evan walked around 10 months old, and Noah around 11 months old. Payton was closer to 13 months old before it was the right time for him. That's ok! Simply being sure that their progress is forward and symmetrical is the most important.

Something else I'd like to address: many people enjoy putting their babies in an "exersaucer." It's fun for the baby, as it keeps them entertained, and it's convenient for the parent so we can get some (much needed and well deserved) space and breathing room. However, this is another device that I believe restricts the freedom of movement and muscle-firing patterns in a negative way. This equipment creates improper postural alignment and can tilt the baby's pelvis in such a position that facilitates incorrect muscle firing and coordination. Babies need to move to develop; and it's through movement that their eyes and ears are stimulated to grow and gain control. This normal function is inhibited by Bumbo chairs and exersaucers.

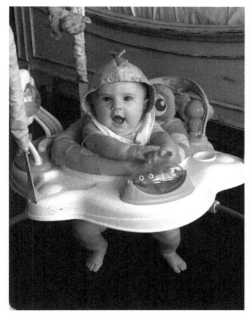 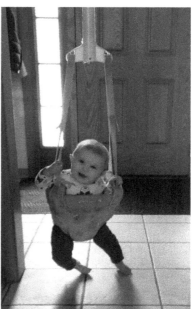

My nephew, Emmett   *My nephew, Asher*

As far as progression to walking is concerned, once again, we don't want to push them into something that their nervous system and muscles aren't ready for. This is illustrated by parents holding their baby's hands leading them forward before they are capable of walking on their own. In these instances, the child has to lean forward and fire other muscles to compensate for that posture. They also tend to move more quickly and in a jerky kind of fashion instead of in a smooth controlled way when they learn to walk independently. Hence, I suggest letting them cruise around furniture, instead of assisting them walking forward while holding your hands at this stage. Your baby is coming to understand his/her own abilities/shortcomings and is teaching his/herself to rely on themselves to problem solve. My pediatrician always said, "never do for a baby what the baby can do for himself." This can be frustrating to watch, but it's also the most beautiful and rewarding experience to watch your child work at something alone and achieve it!

Additionally, I feel I should mention baby footwear. Baby shoes are ADORABLE, but useless! For ideal neurological development and stimulation, babies should be barefoot as much as possible. When learning to walk, barefoot is preferred so they can utilize all the nerve endings and their full foot to balance and gain the sensory input. However, when they begin and will be outdoors/unable to be barefoot, I recommend shoes that are minimalist – as flexible as possible. The brands I found that I loved were Robeez and Bobux. Flexible sole, and squishable if possible! The more mobility the better.

I don't want to come across as neurotic when it comes to allowing your baby to grow. Of course, we want them to roll over. And crawl. And walk. And talk. It's adorable to watch them do these things in our presence. And I would be lying to you if I said I always followed my own recommendations. However, I believe it is critical to let them be the leader and the guide in the process. When we as adults force them into an activity that their nervous system isn't prepared for, the results can be damaging and create what I refer to as "neurological disorganization" as they get older. This is a pattern I commonly see in my children patients who suffer from Attention Deficit Hyperactivity Disorder (ADHD), Autism, Anxiety, and other developmental delays and learning disabilities. I have worked with children with all these conditions with success in helping them, yet, it's best to take a position of support in their journey towards achieving these milestones, so these conditions are less likely to be created in the first place.

Lastly, between 1-8 years of age is where early cortical function and hemispheric dominance begins. I never recommend giving a child an eating utensil or crayons to use before 1 year of age. Usually waiting until 18 months is even more appropriate so as to not force them into dominant handedness before their system is ready. Even at that point, letting them choose which side they wish to use allows them that freedom of movement and choice. There was a time in history where children showing left-handed tendencies would be forcibly pushed to become right-hand dominant which would've been against their genetic determination, once again interfering with their body's proper progression and advancement. Thankfully our culture has matured and no longer "corrects" for left-handedness.

I wanted to provide you with some final encouragement to simply allow natural play to occur. Babies under 2 should rarely, if ever, be allowed to watch television or Ipads/other screens. Screen time is harmful to adults in excessive amounts, so why would we think it's ok to let our babies do this? Now, don't get me wrong, we live in different times now. I am human too, and have absolutely let my kids watch something on my phone or a movie before they were 2. But this MUST be closely monitored. Free play is the most effective way to allow for brain growth, problem solving, and social skills to develop. Electronic toys serve no purpose in these phases. Blocks, colorful toys, squeakers, teethers, puzzles, and books are fantastic tools to create a well-balanced and adjusted child. They learn cause and effect, and object permanence through free play. If something impedes this process from occurring naturally, chiropractic care is often indicated as early as possible to address the nervous system dysfunction before it becomes a greater problem. Remember, as I mentioned earlier, I adjusted and treated all of my kids within hours of their births, and as a gift to my pregnant patients, I always offer to treat the baby for free at the mother's first postpartum appointment. I just know how important it can be to quickly mitigate any birth trauma from affecting their development and reflexes. Not to mention this...

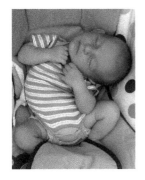

This is my youngest son, Payton, when he was about 4 weeks old. Babies are squishy and flexible, yes, but I'm so glad I was able to adjust him after his nap! They become accustomed to so many cramped positions in utero, it is sometimes necessary to evaluate and treat those imbalances that can lead to problems after birth!

The take-home message here is that the closer we can get to nature and observation when our babies are growing, the better off they will be. Most children will progress just fine on their own with no interventions. They will progress from the discussed phases fluently at their own pace. Whether they walk at 10 months or 15 months does not matter. As long as they are progressing at a pace that is appropriate for them and their motion isn't artificially restricted or forced, they will succeed. This makes your job as a parent much easier, too!

12

It's Easier, and Harder

Most people don't want to be part of the process, they just want to be part of the outcome. But the process is where you figure out who's worth being part of the outcome.

It's simple. I never said it was easy. But it is simple. This process that I have laid out here puts you, as a mother, in a position of being truly conscious and present with every decision you make. You will be one of the few, however, that embraces what you've read here and truly lives it. And guess what? I don't live it 100% of the time either. WE ARE HUMANS RAISING HUMANS. We are <u>supposed</u> to screw up and fail from time to time. In fact, I'm completely sure that I fail at something daily. I just work hard not to live and wallow in that place of failure. I try to embrace the excitement of the journey instead of the struggle—(and this is a lifelong process for me!). While the choices that we as mothers are presented with every day can be overwhelming, you're now equipped with the education and tools to make a more conscious choice. And do you want to know a secret? There's no wrong answer.

A good friend of mine said something with regard to her business goals, and I think it is applicable in every setting. "You will never get it wrong, and you'll never get it done." Assuming you're not abusive or negligent, and provide for the basic needs of your child (food, shelter, warmth and love), you cannot get it wrong. And there is always more that we as parents will want to learn and grow to become better. I know I'm a pretty good mother—and I still go to bed every night wondering what I could've done differently. What I could do better tomorrow? That is the curse of a good mom. It's time to give ourselves grace, love, and respect; and come together and celebrate how amazing we are.

But, instead, many of us choose to complain about the chaos, and feed our babies Cheetos and chicken nuggets because it's easier and what's expected. What baby do you know that eats his/her veggies? What do you think people would say if they knew I co-slept or didn't vaccinate on the CDC schedule? What would a mom friend think of me telling her, "no, I don't use an exersaucer or feed my baby purees." They will think I'm INSANE! I'll come across judgmental and snotty! I may push people away—and while social and cultural pressure is the most difficult obstacle in implementing some of the suggestions I've discussed here, it's not the only challenge you will face. It's sometimes harder to find your "tribe." Your "village" of support and resources. It may be harder to even "google" information that will align with how you want to do things. So, forget it! It's simpler to follow the advice of the masses to blend in and just get through the next 18 years. Hold your breath and power through!

I know I've been here, and to be honest, up until recently, I lived fearfully. Fearful of being judged. So, I hid. I didn't make waves or confrontations. I wanted to look like I had it all "together." My biggest struggle was being real. Admitting to myself and the world that I was a hot mess. Admitting to the world that I'm not perfect. Admitting to the world that I'm still working on my relationship. And admitting that while I practice what I preach, take care of my body and my health, and do a lot of work on myself with self-love, affirmations, meditation, and healing—I still look in the mirror daily and sometimes still pick myself apart. I always wanted to be an inspiration to others, and up-hold an image. But I've learned that the perfect "image" doesn't serve anyone. This fear that we will never be good enough women, mothers, and wives is BULLSHIT that needs to end now. "Good enough" isn't perfection, or pleasing everyone. "Good enough" is simply being who you are.

Repeat after me:

"I AM STRONG."

"I AM EMPOWERED."

"IT IS SAFE TO BE ME."

"I LOVE MYSELF."

"I AM A PHENOMENAL MOTHER."

Feel free to add your own affirmations to this list. I encourage you to begin saying them to yourself daily in the mirror. This was a suggestion from Louise Hay, author of *You Can Heal Your Life* and *Mirror Work*. It has become clear to me that the power behind the words we use regularly is incredible. Even more so with the words we use to talk to ourselves. Don't sell yourself short. You're amazing. You can do this. It's time to stop the self-deprecating talk, and recognize ourselves and each other for the incredible beings that we are. Let's stop the fake, and get real—and start lifting each other up, instead of judging each other on the way down.

I've (mostly) stopped caring about the judgements. Not always—after all, I am still human. But I've been working hard to believe in myself so I can ignore the voices of disapproval/negativity. I don't always advertise my insanity, (except apparently when publishing it in a book!), hahaha! But my choices for how I keep myself sane and my kids healthy are no one else's business but mine, my husband's, and our kids' doctor.

Let's take a humor break and laugh at what motherhood looks like!

"Having a baby is like taking your lower lip and forcing it over your head." -Carol Burnett

"Having a new baby is like suddenly getting the world's worst roommate." -Anne Lamott

"I'm a walking zombie and I think I'm going to be like that for awhile." -Tifanni Thiessen

"A baby changes your dinner conversation from politics to poops." -Maurice Johnston

"You never know when you're gonna get crapped on or when you're gonna get a big smile, or when that smile immediately turns into hysterics. It might be like living with a drug addict." -Blake Lively

"When you have a baby, sleep is not an option. You can't sleep. Even on vacation you wake up at 6:30 a.m." -Jimmy Fallon

"That moment when you go to check on your sleeping baby and their eyes ping open, so you drop to the floor and roll out of the room like a ninja." -Unknown

"Babies are the cutest when they're someone else's problem." -Unknown

"A crying baby is the best form of birth control." -Carole Tabron

"90% of parenting is just thinking about when you can lie down again." -Unknown

"If you want to know what it's like to have a fourth kid—just imagine you're drowning. And someone hands you a baby." - Jim Gaffigan

I LOVE humor. It's how we as humans get through this thing called life. If you haven't figured it out by now, playdates aren't for the kids. They are for the parents. For us to get together and commiserate and share stories, so we can feel like we aren't alone in this world of parenting. It always made me feel better when I would hear that a friend's child behaved similarly to mine! *Thank God, it's not just my kid, or my fault!* We all need that support and community to know that we aren't crazy. This parenting gig is HARD. And I cannot imagine how much more difficult it has been if you're reading this having had your first baby during a pandemic!!! It may be more challenging, but all the more imperative to connect with others during this time. Social distancing won't work long term for a new mother and her baby. It's through humor that we lighten the mood and our hearts to enjoy the process a bit more. If you're looking for an awesome idea for a mom's night out, (when Covid is "over" and we can go out again!), I HIGHLY recommend checking out https://www.thepumpanddumpshow.com/. These women put on a spectacular show and allow you to do what we all want from time to time in motherhood—time away from the baby, with a friend and a glass of wine (or 2, or 3…). They recognize that once you're a mother, girls nights out are a bit different. The bar may not be where you want to be. You suddenly want to talk about spit up, and stretch marks, and nursing pain. With this show you can do it all! They take the raw, realness about parenting and put it into songs and jokes to give you a break!

Here's the thing—we can still connect to normal parenting struggles, while choosing a different route. I didn't start in this place! I just wish that I did—I wish I had someone there ahead of me, holding my hand through this process, letting me know the best practices for myself and my children. But I didn't. I had to do it all on my own. It's ok to be weird. I know that is hard to stomach—but I simply ask that you take my experiences with myself, my own kids, and my patients and their children as a platform to be open to the possibility that holistic living doesn't have to be as crazy as it sounds.

Just because I choose to be conscious about the choices that affect my kids health, doesn't at all mean I don't appreciate parenting memes at their best. 'Cause they are true! And amazing. Have you ever seen the "why is my kid crying?" ones? I'll include some in my next book. Those tend to begin more at the end of the toddler years—oh you have so much in your future!

13

Putting It All Together

Imagine who you want your kids to become... Be that.
-Facebook: The Enlightened Mama

You have the information. You have the tools. The power is in your hands. Now it's your turn. Your choice. Your opportunity to shine. We all have bad days, and we especially have bad days when it comes to parenting. And guess what? So does your baby! Our moods and bodies aren't always grounded and perfectly centered, so why would we expect our children to always act like perfect angels? The goal is not perfection. (*This is coming from an admitted perfectionist*)! The goal is harmony and balance. Mindfulness and presence in each moment. I wasn't there early in my parenting journey. And I really regret that. We can't go backwards—can only move forward. And do the best we can with the knowledge and tools we have at our disposal now.

But, just like Martin Luther King, Jr.'s, "I Have a Dream" speech, I have a dream that mothers will not shame each other for their decisions surrounding their choices regarding their babies. I have a dream that everyone can and will learn about the benefits and drawbacks of everything related to their child's health. I have a dream that we can once again create a village of support for one another. Without judgement. My dream for you is that you are essentially at peace. At peace with yourself, first and foremost. I want you to be happy, fulfilled, and balanced. I want you to feel truly joyful in your own body, mind, spirit, in your romantic relationship, and with the relationship with your new baby! It's completely possible. I've laid out the plan here for you. Your family doesn't need to be destined to have a life of disconnection, confusion and haste. While there will be days of chaos, you can now choose to stay present through each moment. And be the calm within the storm.

I encourage you to get EMPOWERED! You are not weak! <u>You are a WOMAN</u>! You were born to be an amazing and strong human, and now you're raising another person to be just as much a rockstar as yourself. You get this incredible opportunity to watch them develop, teach them kindness, love, and respect, and observe as they create their own path of growth on their journey.

This is not the end of this book, but only a beginning. Parenthood is a journey, just like life. A hypothetical destination is simply an illusion. As we learn and grow more, there will inevitably become new obstacles to overcome. If you haven't heard this parenting quote before, I'll share it with you now: "little kids, little problems—big kids, bigger problems." I can already tell you it's true. But I wouldn't trade my big kid issues for changing diapers again. No part of this process of parenthood is worse, it's just different, and we can be appreciative and grateful for each stage. Because, they really don't last long. Before we know it, that stage you couldn't stand will be over, and you'll be dealing with a new one that will come with its own share of uncertainty and challenges. We may find ourselves missing pieces of what we've now lost. I truly believe that's normal. It's why I cry every time I hear the 2004 Country song "*Let Them Be Little*," by Billy Dean. If you've never heard it, please stop reading, YouTube it, and hold your child tightly while you listen, sobbing. It's cathartic and provides perspective during the tough times! And I promise, I'm usually not a Country fan, so if you aren't either, I assure you it's worth it.

All we can do is our best—and remember the cardinal rules! 1)

Take care of YOU first! 2) Tend to your relationship next. 3) Take care of your babies. Recall from the beginning of this book, this suggestion is not selfish or neglectful. It's simply common sense. Without caring for our needs first, our capacity to provide for others will be diminished or nonexistent.

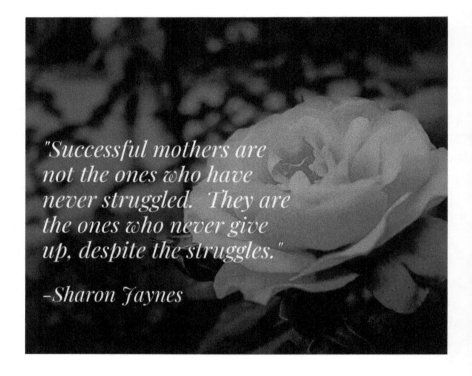

"Successful mothers are not the ones who have never struggled. They are the ones who never give up, despite the struggles."

-Sharon Jaynes

Sending you peace, love, and happiness on your journey!
Until next time!

Acknowledgements

I have so many individuals I can thank, and if I listed them all, I could literally go on forever. My heart is filled with so much love and gratitude for my life and the supportive people that I have in it with me. My parents, Nick and Eileen Artemakis, are amazing people, and provided me a strong foundation of grit and tenacity that has brought me to where I am today. I am so thankful for their encouragement and influence over the years. And I am <u>extra</u> thankful for their time to assist me in editing this book.

To my husband, Jason, and my three beautiful boys: Evan, Noah, and Payton—Thank you for your continued support and understanding of the time and dedication that it took me to write this book. The late nights, the calls, and organization it required to bring this to reality. No words can describe how grateful I am to have 4 amazing men like them in my world. They are my rocks. And I'm thankful for their presence in my life that gave me the experiences to share here that will hopefully influence the lives of so many others.

I would love to also call out our office staff: Sally, Vicki, Kala, Ana, Gretchen, and now Barb, and Michelle. They were always there for me—during my highest and lowest moments through this labor of love. The love, care, and concern they extended me during this last year truly makes me speechless. And so thankful for my newest assistant, Tori, for all her help promoting this work with me!

A special thank you to my dear friend and coach, Jen Zahari. If it were not for her ideas, encouragement, and challenges, I may have still been sitting on all this content waiting for the "right time." She was the most amazing friend and coach through this process I could have ever asked for! Her business and personal growth tips were GOLD and purely irreplaceable. (Highly recommend her if anyone reading needs a personal or business coach: www.jenzahari.com).

Thank you to my Saturday morning "Whoosh" crew: April, Brittany, Dawn, Dorothy, Jen, Kimberly, and Vicki. For all the support, suggestions, and pep talks for my development in so many areas!

I want to extend more gratitude to Dr. Cari Jacobson, Dr. Devon Acou, and Dr. Brad Campbell—for their love and support of me in my health journey now, and in the past. I love all my colleagues in the field of chiropractic and holistic medicine, and you will always hold a special place in my heart. Additionally, one of my biggest mentors, Dr. Tim Francis, taught me most of what I know, and most importantly to always treat my patients with a loving, and compassionate heart.

I would like to thank all of those patients, friends, and family who contributed to this book. Especially Amanda Grace Marcheschi, not only for her contribution, but for also being an anchor of support for me during this time! (You can catch her as "Nurse Dina" on *Chicago Med*!)

A final thanks to all those who did not necessarily contribute, but from whom I learned daily, that provided me more knowledge and understanding to create this manuscript. The lessons they've taught me have been invaluable! And to my new and old contacts and followers in the social media world—it's odd how social media becomes a second family in a lot of ways. Close enough to hold belief in each other no matter what, yet distant enough to not distract from the purpose. I truly appreciate each and every one of them.

I am so deeply filled with humility, love, and infinite gratitude to the universe and everyone in it. I believe everyone we meet leaves some impression on our hearts that causes growth, expansion, and evolution of our spirit. I am genuinely thankful to everyone for everything!

Resources

Most everything listed here you can likely find through the magic of Google. But I wanted to give it to you all in one place, so it would be easier to reference and recall what to look up when you need it.

How to contact/find me:
Email: christymatusiak@gmail.com
Websites: www.christymatusiakdc.com
          www.integratedholistic.com
YouTube: *Dr. Christy Cares*
https://www.youtube.com/channel/UCTPLVPJ6LQnR5HeGVSML25A
Facebook: *Christy Matusiak DC*
https://www.facebook.com/ChristyMatusiakDC
Instagram: *Holisticchristymatusiakdc*
https://www.instagram.com/holisticchristymatusiakdc/
TikTok: Christy Matusiak DC
https://www.tiktok.com/@christymatusiakdc?lang=en

People to know:
Postpartum Doulas – for support and placenta encapsulation
Applied Kinesiology Chiropractic Physicians – icakusa.com
Neuro-Emotional Technique Practitioners – netmindbody.net
Pediatric Chiropractors – icpa4kids.com
Institute of Functional Medicine Doctors – ifm.org

Internationally Board Certified Lactation Consultants – lacationnetwork.com

Milk Donation/Sharing Pages* – facebook.comHM4HBIllinois/ and EatsOnFeetsIllinois/

*These are local to Illinois, you can search to find one local to your area

Finding Your Village Podcast with Amanda Gorman – findingyourvillagepod.com

Bradley Childbirth Method – bradleybirth.com

Hypnobabies – hynobabies.com

Phil Maffetone, exercise heart rate expert – philmaffetone.com

IGT/Low Milk Supply Support Group – facebook.com/groups/ IGTmamas/

Pediatric Dentists – aapd.org

LaLeche League – https://lllusa.org/locator/

Books to check out:

Your Body's Many Cries for Water, by F. Batmanghelidj

The Vaccine Book, by Robert W. Sears, MD, FAAP

The 5 Love Languages, by Gary Chapman

In Fitness and Health, Everyone is an Athlete, by Dr. Philip Maffetone

No Cry Sleep Solution, by Elizabeth Pantley

Helping Baby Sleep, by Anni Gethin, PhD., and Beth Macgregor

The Happiest Baby on the Block, by Harvey Karp

A Couple's Journal: A Year of Us, by Alicia Munoz, LPC

Homeopathic Self Care: The Quick and Easy Guide for the Whole Family, by Robert Ullman, MD, and Judyth Ullman, MD, MSW

You Can Heal Your Life and Mirror Work, by Louise Hay

Biology of Belief, by Bruce H. Lipton, PhD.

Other items for reference:

Berkey Water Filters

Kangen Water

Insight Meditation App
Calm meditation App
Homemade baby formula – https://www.westonaprice.org/health-topics/
childrens-health/formula-homemade-baby-formula/
Documentary – <u>The Business of Being Born</u>
The Institutes for the Achievement of Human Potential – <u>www.iahp.org</u>

About the Author

Dr. Christy Matusiak is a holistically-driven chiropractic physician practicing at Integrated Holistic Healthcare in Wilmette, IL. She works to help others heal through digestive issues, hormonal imbalances, autoimmune conditions, musculoskeletal pain, chronic inflammation, and more. She uses many systems to get a detailed picture of what is going on with each of her patients and focuses on identifying the root cause of these conditions, addressing all areas of their health (physical, nutritional, emotional, and energetic). Dr. Matusiak deeply values the patients she serves to help them and their families live a truly happy, healthy, and fulfilled life.

Dr. Matusiak has been married for 15 years and is a mom of 3 beautiful boys, ages 10, 7, and 5. She remains active with them and is committed to her own health and physical fitness. Dr. Matusiak never gives a patient a suggestion that she does not follow herself! She recognizes that one's journey towards health is multidimensional and always evolving. Through this, she strongly values growth and self-reflection. She believes true health is made up of physical, nutritional, spiritual, and emotional balance. It's her passion to educate the community on how to heal and expand their health holistically. She "coordinates the chaos" in her own life daily, and is excited to share it forward.

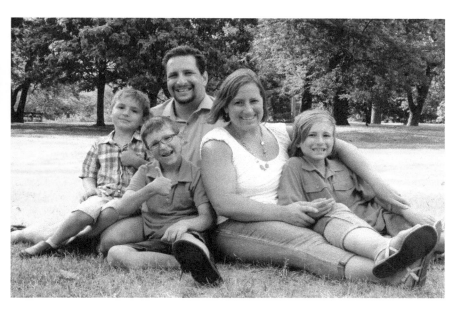

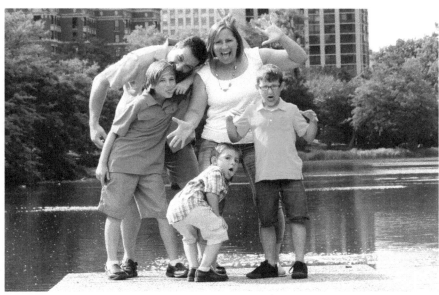

FOL

JAN 1 2 2025

CPSIA information can be obtained
at www.ICGtesting.com
Printed in the USA
LVHW011320060821
694665LV00006B/15

9 781977 243799